S0-ASM-378

The mirror reveals that changes have occurred. What you see disturbs you: a tiny line, or several of them, and what looks like a coming wrinkle, enlarged pores, flaky patches. Cheeks that are sagging a bit; chin muscles that are no longer firm; eyes that are dark underneath, or pouchy. You *do* look different. . . .

For women who have come face to face with these skin problems, hope should spring eternal. Something *can* be done. You *can* look young again. You *can* awaken those dormant muscles, lift them up, help them to smooth out facial and neck lines. You *can* brighten and level out those circles under your eyes. You *can* develop firm and supple tissue, not only on your face and under your chin, but on the backs of your hands also. Not only can you prevent discoloring and "liver spots," you *can* remove them if you already have them.

Here is everything you will ever need to know to keep your skin looking forever young and, most importantly, a remarkable daily regimen that promises instant, dramatic results to every woman concerned with attaining—and maintaining—a radiant, wrinkle-free complexion.

HOW TO KEEP YOUR FACE LOOKING YOUNG

NANCY LANE

PINNACLE BOOKS   LOS ANGELES

HOW TO KEEP YOUR FACE LOOKING YOUNG

An original Pinnacle Books edition, published for the first time anywhere.

First printing, August 1980

ISBN: 0-523-40926-5

Printed in the United States ol America

PINNACLE BOOKS, INC.
2029 Century Park East
Los Angeles, California 90067

To my husband,
our children,
and our grandchildren—
live long and look young.

CONTENTS

HOW TO KEEP
YOUR FACE
LOOKING YOUNG

INTRODUCTION

There was a time when dermatologists and other medical authorities regarded cosmetics as harmful to the skin. Many dermatologists cited what they called hyper- and hypo-allergens in the chemical formulas of various facial creams and lotions. And most of all, the alarm was sounded against the belief that cosmetics would, or could, do anything to better a skin condition or to transform rough, dry skin into velvety, unlined softness. Whereas cosmetics were once designed primarily to alter appearances, they are now being used more and more for medical and physiological purposes, and are intended to not just beautify but to cultivate a more healthful skin condition.

There are cosmetics to make old skin look younger; cosmetics to retard premature aging; cosmetics to heal and ameliorate damaged skin; cosmetics to create nourishing moisture in otherwise parched skin; cosmetics to prevent the harmful effects of the sun; cosmetics to "plump up" tired skin so it camouflages lines and wrinkles, however temporarily; and cosmetics to smooth skin that has become flaky and leathery from prolonged exposure to harmful weather conditions.

Cosmetics have become "cosmedics." What were once only superficial beautifying treats have become skin treatments. Beauty products throughout the world now reflect this change brought about solely by public demand. People today want to be able to buy OTC (over-the-counter) products that will not only make them look good but that will be genuinely good for their skin as well. They demand that their skin both look better and be better.

One might think that cosmetics would have to be classified as drugs to do all this, but such a classification would no doubt be worthless. Virtually anything anybody uses on his or her skin does something to it, whether it's Oil of Olay or imitation mayonnaise. All the major cosmetics firms today are extremely careful to formulate, package, and advertise their products so that they are as safe and effective as they can be. But classifications notwithstanding, many skin-treatment cosmetics are now considered OTC drugs, and one cosmetic manufacturer, Charles of the Ritz, which produces a "Prescribed Skin Care" line, is even owned by a well-known major drug manufacturer, the E. R. Squibb and Sons Company. When Lancôme was ready to introduce its Oil Contrôle skin-care program, the company had six weeks of tests conducted on a hundred people aged eighteen to forty-five at UCLA and at Downstate Medical Center in Brooklyn to find out whether its product could reduce the amount of oil excreted from the skin. Overall, the results showed that the product reduced skin oiliness to a normal level.

The average woman is afraid to consult a dermatologist about a bad skin condition. She would prefer, it appears, to find help in some packaged item she found at a cosmetics counter. And some people with sagging, lined skin would rather do anything than see a cosmetic surgeon. Invariably, they look to cosmetics "discoveries."

Cosmetics firms such as La Prairie, Erno Laszlo, and Payot offer such women a complete line of cosmetics that purportedly produce skin remedies when they are used in a step-by-step program.

It is no small wonder that dermatologists are now looking seriously at specially formulated cosmetics that not only beautify but improve a person's skin.

This book is the result of a public demand. Its aim is to improve your knowledge of the makeup and workings of your skin and how to keep it healthy, not just through use of the right cosmetics but through a concentrated day-by-day program involving at-home skin care, proper diet, vitamins, facial exercises, a positive mental outlook, and everyday living habits.

The results can be "cosmedically" rewarding.

—NANCY LANE

CHAPTER I
WHEN LIFE BEGINS TO ADD A NEW WRINKLE

*Forget about making me beautiful—
just make me look younger!*

a cosmetics customer

If you are under twenty, you, like millions of other young people, are striving to look beautiful. You want to learn everything you can about makeup, hair styles, clothing, and anything else you feel could make you an appealing and attractive person. Unfortunately, in your ardent pursuit of beauty, you may never learn how to preserve the health of your skin and your inherent physical beauty. You may regret this neglect in coming years.

If you are over twenty and under forty, you are learning that whatever good qualities your skin has must be tenderly and precisely cared for if you are going to avoid what television commercials and magazine ads call "premature signs of aging." You are learning firsthand that what goes up must also come down, and that around the age of twenty your body stopped growing and you began aging. You may not be able to see it, but a natural, steady but slow cellular breakdown has begun. The teenage acne is gone, but now monthly pimples sometimes appear. Blackheads are occasional visitors. Your oily skin may make it difficult to put on makeup. Above all, you find you must be more selective about choosing the *right* makeup. Your body is special. Your skin is special. You learn that your skin is a certain type: oily, dry, combination, normal, or whatever. And you also learn that certain skin types require certain types of skin care and cosmetics.

If you are past forty and this side of fifty-five, you are probably well aware that the skin on your face has become a real problem. For years, you concentrated on beauty created mostly by cosmetics, and you tried every new cosmetic that caught your fancy, seeking to highlight or to play down this or that facial feature, flushing or blushing your complexion, making your eyes exotic and your lips dewy and sexy.

You lay for hours in direct sunlight, without wearing a PABA sun-screen. You failed to exercise your facial muscles daily, for fear you would damage your basic beauty. You never drank enough water. Junk foods, rich foods, no foods, a living pattern crutched by vitamins to hype your energy and sex life and to keep you from catching colds. Countless diets led to a jumpy digestive system, a condition exacerbated by, among other things, too much coffee. And you probably coupled a lack of adequate, regular rest with a lack of adequate, regular exercise.

Now the mirror reveals that changes have occurred, almost secretly, yet while you were looking. What you see disturbs you: a tiny line, or several of them, and what looks like a coming wrinkle; enlarged pores; flaky patches; cheeks that are sagging a bit; chin muscles that are no longer firm; eyes that are dark underneath, or pouchy. You *do* look different.

Right away, you think, I'm getting old!

You wonder if your genes, your heredity, got you this way. Or was it worry? You wonder if all this is happening to you because you are you. Thoughts of ag-

5

ing hurt. Deep down, you suspect that you have been doing something wrong. You ask yourself, "What do I do now?"

You shudder at the thought of plastic surgery.

But proper skin care in earlier years could have prevented the development of the conditions described above. For women who have reached the age of fifty and who have come face to face with these skin problems, hope should spring eternal. Something *can* be done. If you suffer from any of these conditions, something *can* be done by you. You *can* look young again. At least, you can look a lot younger than you are. You *can* awaken those dormant muscles, lift them up, help them to smooth out facial and neck lines. You *can* brighten and level out those circles under your eyes. You *can* develop firm and supple tissue, not only on your face and under your chin, but on the backs of your hands also. Not only can you prevent discoloring and "liver spots," you can *remove* them if you already have them. You can create beautiful skin that will make you look as if you are less than thirty.

Looking forever young is not an art. It is a practiced science, a studied regimen. You must work at it day after day. Start out by stopping your search for one cure-all. No one cosmetic product, no one exercise, no one diet, and no one vitamin or rejuvenating potion alone—injected or ingested—will fully correct a lined and wrinkled skin. No one thing alone caused it. Your skin-reclamation program must combine various aids, which together can make you look younger.

Wrinkles and lines do not happen to everyone at a certain age. They happen at all ages. Some people never have wrinkles. Plumpish women seldom wrinkle. Few black women wrinkle. Blondes generally wrinkle quicker than brunettes do. Blonde women with an olive complexion are slower to wrinkle. Many women who live

6

in tropical regions wrinkle early. Some angular women wrinkle earlier. And some sixty-five-to-eighty-year-old-women have no wrinkles. There are reasons behind all of this, and the reasons are more than skin deep.

Octogenarian Mae West, who was always a little on the plump side, was once quoted as saying: "I always stayed out of the sun, and I have taken tender care of my skin every day since I was a young girl." Entertainer Alberta Hunter, who had an unlined brown face when she staged a singing comeback at age of eighty, said: "I never did have trouble with lines and wrinkles. I started early keeping my skin soft with the right creams, exercising my face every day, and eating the right foods. I kept out of the sun, too. I stay away from strong soaps. They dry out your skin. I use a mixture of water and witch hazel. Anyway, black people don't wrinkle quick."

A woman stenographer with an oil company in Alaska, noticing the soft and smooth skins of the region's Aleut females, asked them how they cared for their skin. One of the women told her, "We start when we are young to rub shark-liver oil on our faces. It keeps the cold weather and the strong sun rays from harming our skin."

Some of the cosmetic market's best wrinkle-fighting creams and lotions contain the shark-oil derivative squalane. Orlane's Creme Hydratante Fluide contains the lubricating shark oil, which penetrates the skin rapidly and moisturizes it as well.

SOME CAUSES OF "AGING" SKIN

Aging skin becomes evident when our skin cells are dying faster than our bodies can reproduce them. Prolonged sickness; constant tension, stress, and anxiety;

and prolonged depression all can and do cause skin to age prematurely. Nobody knows exactly why we age, or why some of us age earlier or more rapidly than others. Charles S. Davidson, M.D., of Harvard Medical School, contends that wrinkling is caused by a protein deficiency, which in turn causes the skin to lose its elasticity. Malnutrition—failure to get the necessary nutrients and vitamins—is another possible cause of aging skin. The skin's quality, its texture, and even its moisture content all are directly related to the body's intake of the proper nutrients. Vitamins from foods and supplements, protein, and the essential fatty acids are all as important to the health of one's skin as the very best skin-care cosmetics are. The body needs certain nutrients internally, but it also needs certain nutrients and care externally. We must never forget this. Aging skin can be controlled as chronological age advances. And if these skin conditions have already begun, they can be "tamed".

The woman who is seriously interested in improving her skin condition must at once become critical and discriminating, studying not only advertised betterment programs, but her own physical makeup as well.

Will Lotions Remove Wrinkles?

Remove them? No. Hide them, plump up the surrounding skin, and camouflage them temporarily? Yes. The manufacturers of the anti-wrinkle lotions on the order of Jovan's Wrinkles Away claim that the "removal" action of the lotions is only temporary and mostly for periods "up to eight hours." But I call such products temporary crutches. Why be half safe? A good skin-care regimen, followed regularly on a day-to-day basis with proper diet, exercise, and certain vitamins can give you permanently smooth skin with an all-around glow and appearance of youthfulness, and you will not be required to take eight-hour "jolts" like a drug addict. If your skin is not cared for in this way, and if you continue to use these lotions, chances are that after a while your skin will refuse to react or "plump up" at all.

What Kinds of Vitamins are for the Skin?

Almost all of the vitamins in the B category are helpful to the skin. Vitamin C is great for building collagen elasticin, if bioflavanoids like vitamin P are taken along with the C. RNA/DNA taken daily in 100 mg tablets is also good. PABA, also a B vitamin, in conjunction with folic acid, is excellent for developing good skin. In the chapter "Vitamins and Diets for a Youthful Skin," I shall outline in detail the vitamins that are nutritionally helpful in maintaining youthful skin.

Facial Lines Do Not Always Signal Trouble

Many of us were born with facial lines. In fact, some lines give our faces character and dignity. They identify us. A face without any lines usually looks pasty and lifeless. Our faces reflect our expressions, and, in time, expression lines etch themselves permanently into our faces. But those lines that come about because of worry, lack of exercise and the resultant sagging muscles are a problem and can be minimized.

At times, I have come incredibly close to estimating a person's age by looking at his or her face. But looks can be deceiving. The lines do not always tell. The person without any lines is often older than the person with lines. Even young people can look old if they have the bone structure and features of a desert dweller. The face of a young-bodied female can look like that of Whistler's mother. And many women in their thirties now lay claim to flaky, dry skin with broken capillaries, probably caused by over-exposure to harsh weather and the sun. Many things can make a young face look old and an old face look older.

Stress, Worry, and Anxiety Take Their Toll

These mental states can wreak havoc to the face. They work from within and often become noticeable in strong line etchings on an otherwise smooth face, painting a picture of lingering pain and despair. Medical scientists say that stress is a definite physiological state. But it can stimulate without causing distress and without being unpleasant. In fact, some of us work best under stress. A person watching some of us work under this regular and really necessary stress might say, "You need a rest." Really? A rest would probably give us ulcers, or throw us into a state of worry or depression. Then we *would* be sick. I know that medical findings have shown that constant emotional stress can lead to cancer, but the reports add that this can happen only when the constant stress leads to depression. In contrast to these reports, many other medical people have published reports that questioned this theory.

Constant worry also takes its toll. People smart enough to worry about real things are generally smart enough not to worry too much about them. But there are many of us who worry endlessly about imaginary things, or about things that have not yet happened and probably will never happen. These people worry excessively about matters that a healthy person would dismiss as minor. It is perhaps true that as women get older they have more to worry about and to be moderately distressed about: isolation, financial insecurity, loss of loved ones, and death. There have always been more women than men in mental hospitals, and among those people over sixty-five and in convalescent homes, some eighty percent are women. Let nobody say that women have nothing to worry about.

Author Shana Alexander made the observation in a *Newsweek* magazine article that women working at low-skill jobs quite often worry and feel stress constantly, as they are discontented with their low-level jobs, bothered by their work hours, irritated by the monotony of their lives, and depressed by managers and husbands who don't seem to understand.

We live in an age of anxiety. Anxiety, an unpleasant feeling of tension and apprehension, is closely related to fear. But fear is a natural reaction to some specific thing, while anxiety is a less precise concern about unknown dangers or troubles. When anxiety becomes extreme, we are in trouble. Our endocrine glands and nervous systems, along with various other organs, are affected. After a while, the anxiety begins to show in our faces. Many "worry" lines could more correctly be called "anxiety" lines. An Upjohn Company *Science Information* report said that anxiety can cause insomnia and furrowed brows, and if it progresses into a major depressive disorder, it can lead to a dependence on drugs, alcohol, tranquilizers, or sleeping pills. According to the well-known television medic, Dr. Art Ulene, American women consume three billion Valium capsules each year.

Nutritionists and medical authorities say that certain vitamins and minerals are necessary if the body is to combat stress and anxiety. If your regular diet does not provide these vitamins and minerals, you should take vitamin and mineral supplements. Vitamin A is a stress-related vitamin, but as Dr. Ulene warns, if A is taken by a pregnant women, it can cause toxicity in the unborn child. Other vitamins and minerals related to stress are B-12, B-1, B-3, B-6, C, E, pantothenic acid, calcium, potassium, and magnesium. Later on in this book, there is a list of vitamins that are good for the skin, and other pertinent facts about their effect on our bodies. In addition, there is a list of the kinds of foods that supply these vitamins.

I have found that it pays to eat a bit more food than usual when I am scheduled to face a stressful event. To get ready for the event, I hype up on proteins. I drop about three tablespoons of nonfat dry milk into a large glass of water. Then I add a raw egg and a jigger of brandy. Sometimes I also add a few drops of artificial flavoring, like vanilla, to make the drink taste better. I dump this into the blender, and then into me. It makes me feel able to fight an army.

When we have to cope with something out of the ordinary, our adrenal glands react by spilling adrenalin into our systems, making us better able to face the challenge. But at some time of stress, we could find ourselves tired, due to a lack of the vitamins and minerals that normally stimulate the adrenal and pituitary glands. We need PABA (para aminobenzoic acid), kelp, zinc, and brewer's yeast in our daily anti-stress diets, to be sure. Above all, we should try to put on a happy face each day. A positive, straight-ahead approach will do wonders to banish stress and tension from our bodies and faces.

A good skin-care program will bolster a lot of hopes and brighten faces. But you should also learn to locate your facial and neck muscles. Flex and relax these muscles often. This, too, will chase away a bit of gloom and make your face feel and look a lot better.

UNDERSTANDING THE NEED FOR
SKIN CARE

It is not difficult to understand why any woman would be so concerned about the arrival of facial lines and about enlarged pores and dry, flaky skin. Some women express more alarm over a line or wrinkle than over high blood pressure. After all, a woman's skin presents her to the world. Her face is the first thing her friends, and enemies, notice. Her face is the first thing she studies when she looks into her mirror each day and night.

Beauty is only skin deep, the saying goes. To most women, that's where it all begins and ends. But too often most women just take their skin for granted and never become concerned about it until they feel they are members of the "over the hill" gang. Then it all hits the fan. Their long-time concern over the selection of "warpaint" now gives way to curiosity about healing emollients and flaw concealers.

From Eye Shadows to Shadowing Lines

There was a time when women thought all facial-skin problems could be helped by certain soaps and salves. Antiseptic and rubbing alcohol first, the packaged astringent lotions later. When a wrinkle appeared, a woman merely began to "act her age," and let vanishing creams and powders do the camouflage work. Thinning hair could always be hidden by a hairpiece or hat. Cosmetics went on the face to make one more beautiful. Cold creams, witch hazel, rose water, and gycerine were the "treatment" items. If a facial condition could not be "healed," there was always the cosmetic surgeon;

13

that is, if the afflicted woman had the money and the courage. Many women felt they were keeping their faces younger-looking by having beauticians give them frequent facial massages and mud packs.

But times have changed. Today, women know they can find facial cosmetics to do everything but make new skin out of cloth, if one believes what the advertisements say. But the belief is there. The belief is that cosmetics are not just beautifiers, but helpful aids for the skin. Today's cosmetics contain ingredients known as body nutrients—fruit and vegetable products, vitamins to combat aging, and moisturizing elements that can get moisture from a prune.

For a long time, nutritionists insisted that certain vitamins helped make skin healthful. Vitamin A got such an endorsement. But for a while, many women took so much vitamin A that they developed severe headaches. Medical findings then revealed that too much ingested vitamin A could lead to brain damage. Result: a maximum of 10,000 units per capsule in store-sold vitamin A. But medical science went further and proved that ointments and salves containing vitamins A and D worked well to cure most cases of acne.

Does Dry Skin Really Cause Wrinkles?

Wrinkles develop more easily on dry skin. But the same, and usually hereditary, conditions that make skin dry also make it line and wrinkle. I know some women whose facial skin is so dry that even daily ablutions with Oil of Olay leave it dry. Certain illnesses can cause the body to stop producing moisture. And many angular, blonde, blue-eyed women do not produce enough moisture from early in their lives, leaving them with ultra-dry skin long before middle age. But here again, if the right diets, vitamins, facial exercises, and skin-care cosmetics are used regularly, the person with dry skin should have no fear of developing facial lines.

Can a Cosmetic Say It Will Remove Wrinkles?

Any cosmetic manufacturer should be able to advertise that it can remove anything, if it truly can do so. But the Federal Trade Commission long ago forbade the cosmetic industry from claiming that a cosmetic product could permanently remove wrinkles. What several of the "temporary" wrinkle-removing lotions actually do is plump up the skin to make it appear that the wrinkle has disappeared. But the effect is only temporary, and the lotion ads say so. No cosmetic on the market will permanently remove wrinkles, however.

Then What Good Are the Many Line and Wrinkle Products?

Ultimately, these products are of great help in making the skin softer, less dry, less oily, cleaner, livelier, and more responsive to other bodily reactions that help keep skin young-looking. And this is of great importance to women who neglected to give their facial, neck, and hand skin enough care in their younger years. Some cosmetics help *awaken* dormant skin tissue, just as facial exercises do, and they add nourishing elements made just for a certain skin condition. The new skin-care cosmetics make it easier to apply makeup, too.

What Is Collagen?

The word *collagen* only recently became part of the language of cosmetics, although one cosmetics manufacturer, Germaine Monteil, introduced it years ago as an ingredient in its best skin-care products. Actually, collagen has been with people since they began. Its existence in the makeup of our skin, and the part it plays in maintaining healthy, resilient cellular tissue are of paramount importance to any person seeking to nurture and maintain good skin.

The dictionary defines the word *collagen* as "a fibrous protein found in connective tissue, bone, and cartilage." The collagen used in cosmetics is not ordinarily obtained from humans, however. It is derived from animal tissue, which Monteil only recently stabilized to the point where it could be included in marketable cosmetics. Right beneath our outer skin, or epidermis, the 'true skin,' or collagen, lies in little cushioned pockets on top of the next layer of skin, the dermis. It is a protein substance, and it is what gives our skin its elasticity, as opposed to a sleepy sagginess. These collagen fibers, which connect the skin tissue, can be damaged by age, sunburn, extreme cold, a lack of facial exercise, unhealthful living habits, and a general absence of good skin care. When collagen becomes damaged, expect lines and wrinkles, and all those other little "baddies" that suggest signs of aging.

Do Moisturizers Help Collagen?

Yes, they do. In fact, anything that helps bring moisture to an arid skin helps activate collagen (as vitamin C does with vitamin P). The one thing our skin needs more than anything is water. Twenty percent of our skin is made up of water, and skin without the proper moisture soon begins to dry out, at least the thin stratum corneum does. Most moisturizers protect this skin from environmental blight and reduce evaporation, while softening and smoothing the skin. Moisturizers themselves do not moisturize. They merely seal the pores, causing sweating, thus creating moisture. They work best after the face has been cleaned. Moisturizers can stimulate the dermis, which is less than 1/48 of an inch thick on the face, and their surface sealing action activates sweat glands in the subskin. The sealed-in moisture then softens the skin. Water softens; oil does not.

It is commonly thought that people with naturally dry skins who live in humid environments do not need to use moisturizers. Not so. People born with dry skin need something to *hold in* moisture, to halt its evaporation. Those lucky, darker-skinned people with oily skin are the ones who fare better in humid areas—unless their sebum flow is excessive. But darker women, too, often have dry skin.

What Does Glycerin Do for the Skin?

Glycerin is a great moisturizer. It is a natural humectant, a substance used to preserve the moisture content of lotions. It absorbs moisture from the air, and in cosmetic creams and lotions, stays moist even if the cream or lotion has been exposed to the air. Skin-care cosmetics usually contain glycerol (glycerin) phosphate, which recalls a quote from Dr. Benjamin S. Frank, author of the book *Dr. Frank's No-Aging Diet* (Dell, 1976). Dr. Frank said he had been wondering if glycerol phosphate in cosmetics really could repair damaged cell membranes. If it can do so much good when it is applied, he mused, what could high ingested dosages do? To quote Dr. Frank: "To test this, I began a series of very promising experiments: I swallowed fairly high doses of glycerol phosphate. The results were similar in some respects to nucleic acid therapy! My skin became even tighter and younger-looking, and my near vision, which often deteriorates with age, improved sharply."

The Placenta Extracts and Royal Jelly

Of the skin-care cosmetics with animal-placenta extracts in them, the La Prairie products are probably the foremost. The company achieved world renown for its live-cell placenta formula, which until recent years was administered only in the famed La Prairie Clinic, in Geneva, Switzerland, as a cure for aging. La Prairie's live-cell placenta is, according to the company, obtained from a special strain of black sheep. Then, some years ago, Helena Rubinstein introduced the Tree of Life cream, which was said to contain "extract of human placenta from nature's storehouse of nutrients for the unborn baby."

There has been a widespread impression that Gerovital H-3 contains placenta extract. But all investigation by the FDA has found that Gerovital H-3, pioneered decades ago by Dr. Ana Aslan as the "Roumanian youth treatment and cell rejuvenator," has procaine, the dental anesthetic novacaine, as its active ingredient. It is purportedly a good anti-depressant. Gerovital H-3 was banned in the United States years ago, but its sale was legalized, with a prescription, in Nevada in July of 1977, despite FDA protest. Gerovital H-3 has been tried by millions in Europe, where many persons acclaim the original formula's ability to stave off various aspects of the aging process. Similar praises also come from users of the La Prairie formula, which is a placenta-extract treatment.

As for Royal Jelly, it has long held something of a magical connotation in cosmetics, and has been thought to be able to restore a youthful appearance to skin. It is, however, very nutritious—a mixture of proteins, fats, carbohydrates, water, and trace elements, taken from bees. The actual jelly is a secretion of the throat glands of worker bees, which is fed to the larvae and the adult queen in the bee colony.

When Royal Jelly first hit the market, it lured women by the millions (and still does) to the cosmetics counters. Manufacturers hurried to put it into every kind of facial potion imaginable, with advertisers claiming that the substance would revitalize all skin, no matter how comatose it was. Many cosmetics counters today carry displays of Royal Jelly. Women still buy it, despite infrequent reports in newspapers that the product has not been "proved" to be of any benefit to the skin.

A dozen years ago, a chemist for the state of Michigan's Beauty Counselors, Inc., issued the curt public pronouncement: "Royal Jelly is not even for the birds. It is for the bees. It does nothing for the skin."

For every clinical finding that says bee products are of no benefit for milady's precious hide, there are thousands of women who claim otherwise.

The Great Value of Facial Exercises

One can never say too much about the value of regular exercise for the muscles of the face, the underchin, and the neck. Later on, I shall describe these exercises, step by step. For now, let's get to the importance of these exercises. First, muscles fall into that "use it or lose it" category. If you do not exercise them, they will sag, become flaccid, and seemingly lifeless. Some women are afraid to open their eyes wide for fear of forming wrinkles in their eyelids. But the muscles under the thin eyelids *need* exercise. Even the eye muscles themselves must get daily exercise, like rolling your eyes and looking far askance. Some women believe that keeping the neck craned swanlike keeps away neck lines. The only thing that gets you is a stiff neck. The skin on the throat is truly fragile and thin, but it becomes stronger and livelier as the muscles underneath are exercised. And lines rarely form in the skin of the throat if the neck muscles are snappy from toning. The same goes for the areas around the eyes, forehead, and nose. The areas around the nose that hollow from muscle slackening will fill out if the cheek muscles are put through daily calisthenics.

Do Junk Foods Cause Oily Skin and Acne?

Latest medical reports say no. Most people with oily skin were born with it that way. Usually these are people with tawny skin, dark hair, and dark eyes. And oily skin alone does not promote acne. Hormonal changes, during menstruation and menopause cause pores to clog and acne to erupt. Emotional distress does, too.

During times of emotional stress, use cosmetics to decrease oil production in the pores and antibiotics to kill bacteria that live in the pores. The skin *must* be kept clean. During such hormonal changes, fatty foods *are* harmful. Antibiotics combined with gentle cleansing will keep germs from building up around blackheads, and prevent the formation of spots. Germicidal soaps do no good. If acne develops, the best thing to use on the condition is an acne-treating compound containing retinoic acid, a vitamin A compound that cures acne, expels blackheads, and interferes with the formation of new ones. Benzoyl peroxide is another proven acne and pimple fighter, a compound that produces a mild skin irritation, increases blood flow, and leads to a speedy healing.

How Do "Anti-Wrinkle Lotions Work?

Most of the best-known wrinkle-treating lotions and creams "plump" and puff up the skin. The ingredients awaken otherwise quiet blood cells, making them react with vigor. This is one of the active attributes of the skin-treating regime used by the famed Erno Laszlo Institute. Germaine Monteil promotes this cell-awakening feature in advertising its collagenated creams for the appearance of skin aging.

THE AURA AND POWER OF COSMETICS

Women of the world rely on the magical transformational powers of cosmetics. Synthetic or organic, store-bought, over-the-counter, individually prescribed, door-bought, or plucked from the pantry or garden, cosmetics sell like a life-saving religion. Millions of women depend on cosmetics not just for what they do for the women's appearance, but increasingly for what they do to improve the health of the skin. This enormous reliance is what makes the cosmetics world whirl on its lucrative axis. Cosmetics bring instant joy, however illusory. For every woman who says this or that cream "didn't do me a bit of good," there are thousands of other women who will attest to the helpful qualities of their chosen skin balms, moisturizers, and lotions. Some see virtues in soap, while others profess reasons for not using it. And although soap is not a cosmetic, the cosmetics industry and the soap-making businesses have yearly gross sales in the billions!

Women are more interested in cosmetics than in anything else, it would appear, considering the way they buy countless varieties of them. Vitamins rate a possible second. During the Watergate scandal, congressmen reported that they received more mail from their constituents about vitamins than about the fate of the presidency.

People are interested in anything that will purportedly make them physically better. When a woman buys a bottle or jar of a mixture said to help her facial skin, she is directly investing in a bottle or jar of hope. She is also satisfying a need. People in our society have a daily need for cosmetics to cleanse, beautify, and increase attractiveness.

The U. S. Food, Drug, and Cosmetic Act was passed by Congress on June 25, 1938, calling for truth in advertising. Most cosmetics makers try to adhere to the law, which describes and defines cosmetics thusly:

> 1. Articles intended to be rubbed, poured, sprinkled, or sprayed on, introduced into, or otherwise applied to the human body or any part thereof for cleansing, beautifying, promoting attractiveness, or altering the appearance, and
> 2. Articles intended for use as a component of any such articles; *except* that such term shall not include soap.

Webster defines *cosmetic* this way: 1. "beautifying or designed to beautify the complexion. 2. for improving the appearance by the removal or correction of blemishes or deformities, esp. of the face—*n.* any cosmetic preparation for application to the skin . . ."

Cost versus Quality

Many cosmetics buyers often wonder why a moisturizing cream at the corner drugstore can cost two dollars while a similar product can bring a price tag of fifteen dollars at a swanky downtown department store. "All this stuff's the same," many husbands have huffily told their wives upon seeing a costly new herbal cream the ladies have bought at Sak's or Bonwit-Teller's. "You could have bought the same thing at Cut-Rite Drugstore, and for much less money!"

Is that so? The *same* thing?

Is it possible that Pond's Cocoa Butter skin cream or Johnson's Baby Oil from the corner drugstore is the same as Madame Kumquat's Evening at the Opera Skin Caress Lotion, sold at "better" stores? Hardly. Maybe Pond's and Johnson's could deliver the same results as Madame Kumquat's elixir could. But there again, you would have a difficult time convincing most women cosmetics buyers of that.

Few persons know or consider the lengths to which the maker of a fancier cosmetic goes to bring his or her unique product to market. Chemical research, extensive dermatological testing, high labor and overhead costs, costly machines for precise mixing; bottling, labeling, packaging; massive and costly promotions; shipping; and the privilege of placing it in a store where the clientele cares enough and is affluent enough to demand the very best, and pay for it.

Often, the miracle, break-through cosmetics are first formulated, manufactured, and introduced by makers of costlier cosmetics. Then, after the market has been penetrated by that product, a maker of low-cost products will have his chemists deduce what is in the new product, and how it can be made and sold more cheaply. Copy and cover. Too, there are times when a major, top-line product is marketed through an associate or subsidiary company under a mass-market label, at a price the average woman can afford. In this way, the parent company cleans up all over. Of course, the company would never admit it publicly. But it does happen.

Few major cosmetics makers claim miracle results from their products, unless they qualify those claims. Trained salespeople will tell buyers what the product can **and** cannot do, and will advise that certain results are possible only when the product is used in conjunc-

23

tion with companion items the company also produces.

On the other hand, some of the drugstore items let their labels do all the talking. Such labels state curtly and generally what the product is made to do, and that's that.

But before that Imperial Formula customer is "sold" on the company's special eye cream, at a price somewhere around eight dollars, she understands what the item will do, and under what given conditions. That's why she keeps on coming back for more.

Yet there is hardly a difference at times between that Imperial Formula customer and the housewife who just as religiously returns to her favorite discount store to buy another container of Oil of Olay, resolutely convinced by advertising and trial-and-error use that it is "the mysterious beauty fluid that works with your skin's own natural moisture to ease away dryness." Or, for example, the other women who return to the Thrifty Drugstore shelves to buy Esoterica medicated cream because it "helps fade age spots, freckles, and skin discolorations."

For every woman who plunks down around ten dollars for a two-ounce bottle of Elizabeth Arden's Bye-Lines, there is another who just as joyfully will proffer her less than five dollars for a four-ounce bottle of Jovan's Oil of Mink, because the label says it is a "light luxurious lotion that actually fights the major cause of aging skin." Add the trusting devotees who stick faithfully with low-priced items like Doak's pint-sized Formula 405 and Nivea's familiar dark-blue jar of facial cream. All the customers have reasons why they keep on buying what they feel is good for them.

In the better stores, cosmetics buyers get competent sales help. They get courteous explanations about their skin type, and about which cosmetic items do what and for whom. If a woman who desires a skin toner is allergic to alcohol, the salesperson should know to direct her to one devoid of alcohol, possibly a Lancôme or Orlane product. Some women have found that their skin does not respond well to lanolin, wheat germ oil, or parabens (preservatives and bacteria killers). Consumers appreciate being told alternative products that will possibly satisfy their particular needs. They take kindly to having their individual skin sensitivity, or allergy, discussed and catered to. They usually don't get such personalized attention in stores where cosmetics repose stoicly on shelves and where there is no knowledgeable salesperson in sight.

Many women will buy from unattended counters for a time, as if secretly seeking an ideal wrinkle lotion. After a few disappointments, however, they begin looking for somebody who knows something about skin, and about the many kinds of cosmetics that "do this and that," but which when used "do not do this and that"—somebody who can answer a simple question like "How does one develop wrinkles?" or "Do wrinkles come and go?" A customer might never get the answers at an unattended cosmetic shelf, or even at most drugstore counters.

What *is* a wrinkle, really?

Webster defines *wrinkle* as "1. a small ridge or furrow in a normally smooth surface, caused by contraction, crumpling, folding, etc. 2. a crease or pucker in the skin, as any of those caused by aging, frowning, etc."

Germaine Monteil, the first cosmetics company to introduce 100 percent pure, stabilized, soluble, unlinked collagen, says this about wrinkles:

"As aging progresses, soluble collagen diminishes in the skin. The collagen molecules become inflexible due to the crosslinking. This crosslinking causes the colla-

25

gen to become inelastic. This inflexible and inelastic collagen is responsible for wrinkles and creases."

A woman's skin is all her own. What she puts on it and what reaction she gets from it are her own business. It's her own beauty she has to build, modify, and project. Her dreams and sense of trust should not be dashed by someone claiming that what she is using does no good. Again, it's her own skin.

But is it all that simple? Surely not.

Behind all that trust in cosmetics with fancy names and claims, the woman buyer is motivated by hope. Whether or not anyone has ever told her, she knows that all things change, including her skin. Every creature ages, and she never forgets that. She knows her face changes, for whatever reason. Her mirror tells her so. And when her spirits and physical strength are low, she is aware that her face reflects those conditions.

What is foremost on her mind throughout her life is what she should do about her face to offset those facial changes, to slow some of them down, to hide them, or to prevent them altogether. She wants to know what is right for her skin: what to do to treat those encroaching lines, puffy pouches, worry creases, scaly flakes, greasy shines, and those wretched wrinkly conditions.

To start, she should know about her skin itself.

CHAPTER II

THE UNIQUE HUMAN SKIN

I am resolved to grow fat and look young till forty, and then slip out of the world with the first wrinkle and the reputation of five-and-twenty.

John Dryden, *The Maiden Queen*

Not every human being has the same type of skin. At times, it would appear that everyone's skin is the same, but that is far from true, no matter how much some cosmetics advertisements seem to propagate the notion that what's good for Suzie's skin is equally good for Sally's. Chances are, Suzie's skin reacts against metallic mercury, alcohol, lanolin, acetone, and preservatives used in certain cosmetics, while Sally's skin accepts anything. It is truly pathetic how many women run into difficulty buying skin-treatment products because they do not know their own skin types. But how *are* they to know? Skin care and skin types are not subjects generally taught in public school.

There are nearly two dozen skin types. Most of us have one of a dozen of these types. Despite these numerous skin types, however, most of us have skin that falls into one of three basic categories: normal or combination, oily, dry. Some women like to boast that they have "sensitive" skin, as if all skin were not sensitive to

27

some degree. But a truly sensitive skin tends to be dry. It follows that many people with "sensitive" skin also fall into the category of those persons who do not know their skin types.

One of the most simple tests for checking your skin type is to take a short piece or strip of cellophane tape and place it (glue-side toward the skin) across the bridge of your nose, with the ends sticking out and covering portions of your cheeks. Let it stay on for a few seconds, then gently remove it. Hold the tape under a bright light. If it has picked up a lot of little white dry flakes, your skin is dry. If there are no flaky particles on the tape, and if it has a wet-looking sheen, your skin is oily. If you have a combination, or what is generally regarded as normal skin, the tape will show the dry flakes from the cheeks, and have the wet sheen from the area around the nose. This test works best about an hour after you have cleansed your skin thoroughly. Do not conduct the test during times when your skin is reacting to hormonal changes brought on by menstruation or menopause. During such times, the skin reacts abnormally.

All skin is analyzed best when looked at under the lighted magnifying glasses some makeup experts use. A pioneer in the use of such glasses was the late Eddie Senz, who for years was acclaimed as one of New York City's East Side makeup experts. Senz was a facial genius for actresses Jayne Meadows, Rita Gam, Lena Horne, and women stars of the Metropolitan Opera. After he had studied each client's face carefully under the glass, he would mix an entire cosmetics line for the client. When the client wanted more of her individual skin-care products, Eddie Senz's company would make it for her. Each woman's skin formula was kept in the Senz file, with a list of the woman's skin texture, condition, and allergies, plus the customer's skin absorption ability and notes telling which components blended best on her skin.

But every woman cannot go to such lengths to learn about and treat her skin. It is hardly easy for the average woman to get her skin classified accurately according to age, sensitivity, balance, and type. Even learning whether her skin is allergic to something can be trying.

Speaking of allergies, we are not always born with them. Some of them get worse as we grow older. Most often, the woman who breaks out in a mild rash (or a severe one) after using a specific cosmetic product instantly blames that product. But it can hardly be the cosmetic itself. It could be that a certain ingredient in that cosmetic product is to blame, a little gremlin that works well on the skin of most cosmetics users, but that acts up when it touches the skin of certain women. The job is to find that particular ingredient. Start by looking at the contents of the products. Chances are, the culprit is one of the best skin softeners in use—lanolin. Or it may be the parabens (preservatives) in the product. Does it contain alcohol? Since it is so difficult to learn just which substance is the allergy-causing culprit, short of going to a dermatologist, most women merely test the product by placing a bit of it on the insides of their arms, and leaving it there overnight. If there is no redness the next day, the coast is clear. That is probably the best and easiest way to test for allergies. The tests that dermatologists use for allergies cost a lot and often take weeks.

Seldom will one encounter allergy-causing substances in skin-care and skin-treatment products. Most makers of skin-care products try hard to set the highest standards, not just to be lawful, but, more important, to market a satisfying product that will create a lasting and profitable reputation for them. More often, allergy complaints come from people who use ordinary

29

makeup products. But makeup manufacturers labor assiduously to exclude reactive ingredients from the items in their lines, too. Today, you find many cosmetics makers producing skin components that do not have scents, because ingredients in perfumes sometimes cause skin irritation. Makeup, again, is usually for the purpose of creating an image not necessarily for skin health. Makeup is good for hiding and highlighting, for concealing and "playing down," and increasing individual beauty. Skin-care cosmetics do more. They make the skin healthful and youthful. Makeup is psychological. Skin-care is for real.

Bleach creams often awaken allergies. They should be used with care. Some of them contain mercury, the quicksilver element that is often irritative to the skin. Hydroquinone has been substituted for the condemned hexachlorophene, but hydroquinone can also cause painful skin irritation in cases where an allergic condition may already exist.

Cosmetics should never be hastily blamed for allergic reactions that could have been caused by some other external or internal conditions.

SOME COMMON SKIN TYPES

Normal Skin

It is rare to find normal skin. Its texture is fine, unusually smooth and elastic, and it has no enlarged pores, pimples, or blemishes. It shows no evidence of oiliness or lack of moisture. Women with normal skin attest to doing little to enhançe, correct, or sustain their skin condition. And they admit that they have spent very little time in the sun. But such skin *is* a rarity. Unfortunately, most of us fall into one of the other categories.

Problem Skin

This kind of skin is the opposite of normal skin. Problem skin is generally rampant with clogged pores, unwanted blemishes, and minute eruptions, making the woman feel that her skin condition is a ghastly carryover from the pimply teenage years when Clearasil was used by the tub. This kind of skin requires constant attention, precise care, and a treatment regimen that does not vary until the condition improves. Above all, panic should not dictate use of a crazy assortment of cosmetics. The danger is that one item will clash with another and further inflame the skin. Frequent cleansing, disinfecting, and drying are required. The person with problem skin should never try to buy every kind of treatment advertised, in the hopes that her condition will be alleviated more quickly if she uses a touch of this and a touch of that. She should seek advice from qualified skin consultants when she is in doubt about a product. In the chapter on skin regimen, there are specifics on those cosmetics that will provide surface help for the person with problem skin. Other sections of this book tell about other aids as well.

Oily Skin

This condition appears to be very similar to problem skin. It is characterized by enlarged pores, frequent blackheads, and a perpetual greasy film over the face. The open pores appear more coarse and pronounced, giving the skin the look of an orange peel. All this is due to the excessive flow of sebum.

Lancôme markets a grand three-item product to control this oil problem. Called Contrôle de Lancôme, it consists of a priming cleanser, a regulating liquid, and a

31

maintenance cream, which, when used according to directions, is supposed to reduce surface skin oil to a more normal level and help keep it that way. Otherwise, clean the skin frequently, and use facial masks and packs to tighten the skin and keep the pores free of grit and grime blockages that can cause blackheads and infections. Naturally, the sebum flows more freely, but the skin will maintain its good health. Problems from oily skin are usually only temporary anyway. In the long run, the oily skin will be the last to show lines and flaky patches. It's always easier to keep an oily skin supple and soft. But do not let some ambitious cosmetics salesperson scare you into buying everything on the market to "stop all that oil." Looking under a magnifying glass at the enlarged pores of an oily skin *will* scare you. Orlane came out some time back with what it called a skin scanner, which magnified a person's skin surface many times. It made oily and problem-skin areas look like a ravaged countryside with deep gullies, hilly risings, scaly plateaus—bristly, greasy, and generally alarming.

Dry Skin

Dry skin is "in." You've simply got to have it, it would appear. With all the moisturizers now on the market, one would think that all women have dry skin. Dry skin is characterized by its fine but tight texture. It lacks moisture and oil, and has a tendency to wrinkle, making many women feel old age is at hand. The condition is more apparent around the eyes and mouth, causing lines at the corners and verticle lines on the upper lip. But these lines, like dry skin itself, can also be a hereditary trait. You just have to moisturize more, lubricate more, and exercise the facial muscles more. Increased intakes of lecithin and cod-liver oil also will help greatly.

Combination Skin

Combination skin displays both dryness and oiliness in various places. The oily areas usually are found where sebum flow is normally at its highest—on the forehead, chin, cheekbones, and nose. Dryness usually is found around the sunken or lower sections of the cheeks and the areas around the outer part of the eyes. Naturally, different kinds of treatment are necessary for each area.

Sensitive Skin

There are reasons that some skin is called sensitive. Broken capillaries abound, running off in many directions like little red rivulets. Rashes break out at the least whisper. Each tiny pimple threatens to become an ugly blotch. Lines form in groups. The sun irritates so-called sensitive skin, for the sun is generally the chief cause of such skin conditions. Harsh cold during winter months can make sensitive skin react badly, too. Those capillary eruptions can be removed by a dermatologist. And other conditions can be helped by moisture-trap cosmetics, but be sure to use those containing a PABA sun screen and adequate skin-protective oils. Even then, it helps to wear brimmed hats and sunglasses in the sun, to shield the upper cheeks and the areas around the eyes from harmful ultraviolet rays.

ENVIRONMENT AFFECTS SKIN

Where you live does make a difference as far as your skin is concerned. And where you live can affect and change your skin, making these effects more noticeable on exposed areas such as your face, neck, and hands. The longer you live in certain locales, the worse off your skin will be.

Tropical areas can be very harmful. Just a few months in the open in such areas, without protective sun screens and without skin-protective moisturizers, often causes your skin lasting problems. Blood vessels rebel, crack, and break; the skin reddens; and the outer skin hardens, since it has developed something of an armor to protect the more vital inner layer.

Cold and windy areas also contribute to a breakdown of the outer skin. Protective measures should always be taken. In fact, women who expose facial and neck skin to the elements must go to greater lengths to fortify their skin and protect it.

And those happier souls living in forever-summer areas are not out of danger, either. With more and more cars on city streets, and all kinds of pollutants filling the air, it is easy for women with dry skin to develop itchy skin. The impurities in the air make the skin break out with irritating spots, and cause the skin to lose its elasticity. Again, the prevailing regimen should be a liberal application of moisturizers massaged into the skin, followed by a good sun-screen lotion. Cleansing is paramount under such conditions, and often, with your preferred skin cleanser or a mild soap, like Neutrogena.

NOTHING CASUAL ABOUT THE SKIN

Some people tend to be quite casual about their skin. These same people may regard their skin as a mere layer of flesh that nature designed simply to hide and protect vital bodily organs underneath, like a heavy garment to protect one from the cold.

Actually, the skin is a living, breathing entity—a working blanket of delicate machinery. The top layer of the skin is called the *epidermis*, and the layer directly beneath the top layer is called the *dermis*. Under that, and linked with the other layers by fiber tentacles, is the *subdermis*, or *hypodermis*. Covering the first layer is a thin covering of flaky dead cells that are always shedding, or peeling, off because of the rubbing action of clothing or massaging towels. A nasty sunburn can cause this thin outer layer to peel. But the epidermis also has a regenerative ability, and it can replace the ever-peeling surface veil. It also protects the lower dermis from many surface dangers. The dermis needs protecting, for it contains blood vessels, nerves, and fatty tissue, and it has sweat and oil glands, along with countless hair roots. From these roots, hair pushes its way through cell shafts to the outer perimeters of the epidermis. The hair roots are nourished by a constant coating of sebaceous oil, making the growing hair healthy and glistening. Although we cannot always see these growing hairs, they are there, however tiny and wispy, like an incessant blanket of soft, diaphanous fuzz. On some of us, they are quite obvious, and present constant plucking problems. Painful ones at that.

Eyebrow hair is stronger in texture, bolder in color, and more pronounced. But there are always countless hairs growing over the other parts of the face as well.

35

Pluck one hair out with a tweezers, and another hair shortly replaces it.

Some of the tiny holes on the surface of the skin do not contain hairs. But inside those tiny holes, mistakenly called pores, are oil glands that send forth oil films that some say cause blackheads to form on the skin surface. Dermatologists differ on whether or not daily cleansing of the surface of the skin will prevent blackheads from forming. We shall get to these opposing claims later. Nothing can close these tiny holes and cap off the oil excretions the way one would cap an oil well.

Actual skin pores are so small that it takes a good microscope to see them. In some way, they act as waste passages in the skin, in that they permit the body to give off perspiration through their channels. The pores also exude natural body oils to lubricate and nurture the outermost skin surface. It's easy to see why the pores must be kept clean.

There are substances that can penetrate the skin's surface and get into the body, affecting the dermis. Antiseptics can. Liniment can, and some rather strong astringents can. But our cosmetic industry has never come up with a cosmetic that could plumb the depths of the second-layer dermis and change it. Moisturizers and collagenated cosmetics have their claims, but in no way can they alone rebuild the fatty tissue that comprises the lower layer of the dermis and plumps the skin to make it smooth and appealing. Nor is there a cosmetic that can re-plump the fatty dermis in older women. As a person ages, the fatty dermis becomes a bit thin in spots, hanging loosely, its protein and collagen disconnected, and its cells broken down. The result of all this is that frowns, grimaces, scowls, and grins eventually begin etching lines and wrinkles into the face. Inside-out treatment becomes necessary.

No matter how old a person is, the skin is a never-resting chemical factory. It manufactures keratin, which is a component of the skin, fingernails, and hair, and melanin, which gives our skin its color. There are special DNA enzymes that "tell" the skin when to work and when not to work, and how much work to perform. The skin even produces its own bacteria, antibiotics, and histamines. The antibiotics fight off toxins, and the histamines control blood-vessel dilation.

In addition to replacing normal tissue, the skin also is able to heal and clean. When there is a cut on the skin, the skin heals itself. When there are severe abrasions, the skin heals itself then, too. It cleanses itself by expelling impurities, even when we are asleep and no matter what is on our face. And fortifying keratin makes the new skin durable but resilient.

Healthy skin has a constant covering of a substance that feels like a mild witch hazel or glycerine water. It is like an emulsion of water and oil, and it provides a certain but limited protection for the surface of the skin. It is understandable why we are often cautioned against taking too many baths and showers with strong deodorant soaps. The fear is that we will wash away this important surface substance. Indeed, if the skin were not permitted to "do its own thing" in renewing this emulsified protective film, it would become dry and leathery. Its normal moisture would surely disappear.

This protective film is called *sebum*. It is a natural oil that lubricates the skin. Sebum is turned out by the *sebaceous* glands, in the second layer of the skin, and it rises to the surface through microscopic openings called pores. When the sebum flows properly, our skin is soft and pliant. If the glands are overworking, the surface skin will become oily, the pores oil-logged. On the other hand, if the sebum is not flowing normally, the result can be tight and brittle skin, with a surface as dry as an arid riverbed. Sebum is programmed by nature to flow more freely during our adolescent years, causing many teenagers to seek any solution that will halt or slow the sebum flow. As teenagers mature, the sebum flow slows down, and in older people it sometimes stops flowing altogether, causing millions of women to head for cosmetics counters to find emollients and moisturizers to stimulate better sebum action while lubricating the already seemingly parched skin.

Vigorous cleaning will usually wash away the results of good sebum action. It then takes three hours for the sebum to rise once again to the skin's surface. People with aging skin should use moisturizers that lubricate and hold in natural moisture, but that diminish the effects of dry cold and pollutants as well.

Sebum flows more freely and collects more often on a person's forehead, and more so in males than in females. For some unexplained reason, sebum flows less in older women, particularly women of very fair complexion. Women with darker skin often enjoy good sebum action well past fifty. In winter months in colder climes, women tend to notice that less sebum flows, as if it retreats, shivering from the cold, thus leading to drier skin. This sudden dryness spurs many women to use massage oils, petroleum jellies, cold creams, and other greaselike substances on the chapping, splitting skin, not knowing that the skin's dryness in cold weather is more often caused by a lack of moisture than by the cold. By contrast, in summer months, the skin tends to sweat easily, and therefore gets moisture. Some women don't sweat, or perspire, too freely, though. It is not hard to understand why so many women today have turned to suitable moisturizer cosmetics.

Yet, in spite of all the preparations available, at prices within reach of most people, many women still do not care for their skin properly, and permit the surfaces to crack and crease, line and wrinkle, as if nature is bound to have her way no matter what. Maybe it is caused by laziness brought on by the many cares and worries of the day, or perhaps it is because they just do not know exactly what to do and never were adequately and simply told what to do.

One woman asked me what she should do about the "little lines" in her face. She wanted to know if I thought very much of the cosmetic Line Tamer, which she was using. She quickly added that much to her dislike, the product left a whitish residue. I started to tell her jokingly not to worry about it, that in every twenty-eight days the skin renews itself anyway, and that maybe after that time she would have a new unlined epidermis. But then I realized that it was no joking matter. If unlined skin did appear every twenty-eight days, there would be no need for any man or woman to worry about lines. I had to be serious. The lady was desperately serious, and she wanted help. She was like millions of other women who search everyday at cosmetics counters, hoping to find something that will transform an unsatisfactory facial condition into a satisfactory one.

My answer did not denigrate Line Tamer, although I did tell her that not even the best anti-wrinkle cosmetic can provide plumping that will last over a twenty-four period. Some do not leave whitish residues, however; and that is how I approached answering the query.

Many women want to buy beauty and sex appeal since they feel they were born without it. And there are women who feel that any thin facial line or any possible wrinkle means vanishing beauty and youth. For most men, lines are not really a bother. But for some men, wrinkles are as scary as they are for women. So, many women and men cosmetics buyers secretly seek to buy yesterday's youth.

39

Mental stress, which often causes skin disorders, can be caused by skin disorders, too.

Most line-hiding and skin-plumping lotions are excellent for smoothing out the rhytides, or fine facial lines, in the face. The resultant appearance is a smooth, velvety, healthful-looking skin. But this peach-glow look will last only for a short time. After all, cosmetics are only temporary. How wonderful it would be if consumers could buy a bottle that would keep their faces smooth until they were eighty, a la Mae West!

Only a cosmetic surgeon can adequately "lift" a face so that there will be somewhat lasting results. Such an expert surgeon will be able to remove and redistribute skin and surgically reinforce dormant facial musculature.

Kurt J. Wagner, M. D., and Gerald Imber, M. D., in their explicit book *Beauty by Design* (McGraw-Hill, 1979) say that aging and loss of skin elasticity can be caused by over exposure to the sun, a topic that will be treated in full later on in this book. Alcohol, poor nutrition, and an inadequate amount of sleep and exercise can also hasten sagging and aging, say the doctors, who add that this unfortunate fiber deterioration represents skin changes that "can be reversed only by the surgical face lift." But these expert surgeons explain in their superb book that "it should be made clear that the elasticity and general health of the skin are in no way improved by undergoing such surgery. What is taking place is simply removal of a portion of the stretched-out skin and a redraping of the remaining skin so as to make the loss of elasticity less noticeable. The skill of the surgeon is thus directed at reducing, tightening, and smoothing the skin, and generally at helping to overcome the effects of life style, years, and gravity, upon the face."

In one of its customer questionnaires, Clinique Laboratories posed the query: *Is it true that at present there is nothing to be done for skin sag?* Clinique's answer: "Surgery is the only true help at this moment in cosmetic history."

Millions of women, however, would rather find another answer to the problem of sagging skin, and, like so many women with line and minor wrinkle problems, they look to marketed cosmetics and skin-care and skin-treatment regimens, no matter how temporary the effects. No-surgery face-lift exercises are becoming as popular as magazine diets. Mega-vitamins, especially vitamins having to do with tissue-building and the triggering of enzymes, are the vogue with many women who feel their bodies are going through various changes reflected in their faces. RNA/DNA are better understood, and foodstuffs, especially tropical fruits and herbal derivatives, are selling to people trying to stave off the effects of onsetting age. And women of all ages are bicycling, rowing, jogging, skating, swimming, bending, walking, and putting not only their bodies but their faces through all sorts of isometrics. Somehow, by reading, watching television, and listening to radio, they have come to the conclusion that good physical health, motivated by a purposeful and positive attitude, can be achieved and maintained by a combination of these and other things. Most of them do not know or understand the intricate and still somewhat nebulous workings of the human body, but they are starting to see their bodies as fine machines that can be kept in working shape with attentive care.

One Beverly Hills woman I know, who has had four eye-pouch lifts, called blepharoplasty, confessed to me that she smoked heavily in her younger years, consumed liquor daily, and was a virtual sunbathing fiend, all of which made the skin beneath and above her eyes show early signs of muscle fatigue, thinning, and stretching. "I had begun to show aging signs, like lines and crow's feet around my eyes before any other part of my face showed them," she said. "Don't call them laugh lines, because I was never one to laugh very much. But the lines were there. I had one eye lift, then two years later the lines and pouches were back again. I've had four, and I shall not have another, no matter what the doctors tell me about there being no chance of nature's giving me any new tissue under my skin where they took out that pouchy tissue." The lady said she now "babies" her skin, using selective cosmetics to give the skin around her eyes a seemingly youthful appearance, and, she added, "I eat the right foods, take the right vitamins, and get the right exercise. And I am happy."

Aside from the effects of too much alcohol, too much sun, too much smoking, and too little exercise, there are certain built-in factors that assault youthful, elastic tissue and cause facial lines and wrinkles. These factors, at present, can't be reversed, reduced, or avoided by any plastic surgeon. Research shows that good health habits in one's young years can delay or temper the effects of aging later on. I say these factors are "built in" because gerontologists and biologists have found that no matter how we take care of ourselves, Mother Nature has prescribed before birth our individual "lasting" abilities, through a possibly set period of time.

Dr. Bernard Strehler, of the University of Southern California's biology department, found that old tissues are unable to manufacture ribosomal RNA (ribonucleic acid), which is vital in the synthesis of new proteins, without which a cell cannot divide or survive. He likened the RNA/DNA process to a factory, with RNA being the work site on an assembly line where body parts are being put together according to a blueprint—the parts here being amino acids and protein. Dr. Strehler believes that the body's genes (whits of DNA that dictate differences and characteristics) for RNA are "iced" after a set stage in each individual's physical or chronological development, and are then turned off, as if by an unseen hand when Mother Nature says the time has come. Growth stops. This is fortunate, contends Dr. Strehler, for if the turn-off did not take place, we would keep on growing like a giant cancer. Without the built-in turn-off, we'd probably all grow to be jolly green giants. But the turn-off happens to everyone, the production of new proteins stops, and aging begins. Not at forty, not at fifty, but usually around the end of our teens and the beginning of our twenties. It seems cruel and mean of Mother Nature to make aging begin as soon as growth ends. But Dr. Strehler says it is the hope of medical science to find ways to develop certain viruses that would reactivate the RNA genes, which in turn would make certain body cells produce healthy, elastic tissue.

Stanford University's Dr. Leonard Hayflick, in a March 1973 Los Angeles *Times* article on aging, said the key to aging lies in the genetic information stored in the cell, the DNA concertmasters that tell RNA what to do, and when.

"Normal cells," said Hayflick, "seem to have a definite limit to the number of times they can divide, and this fact may or may not have something to do with aging."

Hayflick said he feels that the body has a specific gene that directs a blueprinted program for aging, and at a certain stage of life, certain body cells are told to slow down their reproduction, and finally to cease their building program altogether. "One example of this might be menopause," he explained, "which occurs at a certain time in all women's lives, give or take a few years." Hayflick said his tests of cell cultures in his laboratory found that normal cells replicate about fifty times before running out of steam and dying. But, he points out, "I don't think we age because our cells no longer divide. Rather, we age because of functional changes that occur in the cells *as they divide.* Around the thirty-fifth doubling, we begin to see changes that herald the appearance of aging."

Medical science believes further that as our body cells diminish in capacity, we become more susceptible to ailments and diseases, and more likely to develop lines and wrinkles. The immune system begins to break down, and "mutants" develop. Some cells may not recognize these new cells as "self" and may begin to attack them as "non-self."

On May 13, 1979, Dr. Roy L. Walford of UCLA was quoted in a Los Angeles *Times* article by George Alexander as saying that he and other biological researchers had concluded that the set of genes involved in identifying "non-self" molecules and destroying them, thus creating a strong bodily immune system, is called the "main histo-compatibility complex."

These genes manufacture enzymes, said Dr. Walford, that "read" the DNA (deoxyribonucleic acid) in a cell. They also can recognize small errors in the DNA of "self" cells, and can snip off the damaged or erratic parts and restore the molecules to its proper biochemical condition. Dr. Walford revealed his findings in a lecture he gave at the National Institute of Aging, in Bethesda, Maryland. He added that this recognition of the body's "repair crew" of genes will help medical scientists retard aging in human beings.

Earlier, Dr. Walford had said that "the aging program could be contained in just a few of these genes. I would look for these genes on those chromosomes that are involved with the immune system. One of these is H2 (the chromosome which is thought to control the

44

rejection of skin grafts, and even transplants, from other donors)." The scientist pointed out that diet and body temperature affect the immune systems and possibly influence the aging process. Laboratory tests have shown that mice live longer when their caloric intake is sharply reduced. One test disclosed that young mice fed only seven calories a day plus certain vitamins even looked younger than animals of the same age fed the ordinary fifteen calories and no vitamins. Echoes Dr. Walford: "Undernourishment, not malnourishment, is the answer. It has to be good nutrition."

Each of us began life as a single cell, one fertilized egg. By the time we are twenty, that one cell has multiplied into 100 trillion cells—a grown-up human. But as these cells die off, we age. As cells get sickly, so do we. Even the cells that are well age.

Each human cell contains about 50,000 genes— enough to make another complete human being just like you. DNA (deoxyribonucleic acid), the nucleus of each cell, is also your blueprint. Biologists believe that the genes program cells for aging, after a predetermined number of divisions. Scientists, trying to alter DNA's program, are literally trying to make dying cells "born again."

Through what is called recombinant genetics, medical scientists have already found ways to insert strands of DNA into bacteria, to manufacture insulin, making it possible for the first time to produce insulin injections composed of human pancreatic juices. Before that, every insulin product was derived from animal pancreases—the same process and product used in current "live cell" skin-rejuvenation cosmetics and "youth-replenishing" therapy. Researchers at the University of California-San Francisco and Genentech, Inc., have already synthesized the hormone required for growth, using cultures from human pituitary glands. This synthesized hormone may make it possible for people afflicted with dwarfism to grow to normal size.

As scientists try to synthesize DNA in body and skin cells, they know, too, that when they find the agent that "turns off" normal cells they also will be on the threshold of the discovery of the causes and possible cure of cancer. Aging will probably not be stopped, but it may be slowed down.

Using certain cell cultures, Joan Smith-Sonneborn, at the University of Wyoming, has extended by fifty percent the lifetime of the single-cell creatures *Paramecia tetraurelia,* reported *Newsweek* magazine on August 20, 1979, adding: "First, she dosed them with ultraviolet light, which actually reduced their life expectancies. Then she subjected them to longer-wave ultraviolet or 'black light,' and this delayed the aging process. Smith-Sonneborn speculates that the first dose damaged the DNA in the cells but switched on a natural repair mechanism in the genes. The black light then eliminated the harm caused by the ultraviolet, while allowing the repair process to mend or prevent other damage in the genes. Researchers now hope to find ways to overcome the damage of age in other types of cells."

Through all this intense study into human genes and their functions, scientists are learning more about how we come to be the individual human beings we are and what can be done to "correct the mistakes" that send us to doctors again and again, and that make us retreat from our mirrors.

It is no accident that cosmetics products today are made more and more with substances that can affect change and correct bodily manifestations and conditions that were often dictated by our own genetic makeup. La Prairie's live-cell therapy, developed from anti-aging treatments begun at the La Prairie Clinic in

Geneva and now embodied in the line of La Prairie skin-treatment cosmetics, concentrates entirely on such genetic skin conditions, as does the rejuvenation therapy GH3 of Dr. Ana Aslan.

We are all learning the importance of a good diet and a good vitamin-regimen to maintain good skin health and to combat all signs of aging skin. We are learning more and more what to eat and how much, and how exercise can help improve the body and skin. We are learning the danger of excessive eating, excessive drinking, excessive smoking, excessive sun, and excessive disregard for our skin. As bizarre and scary as it may seem, all this talk about genes, cells, DNA, RNA, immune systems, aging, allergies, nutrition, and the like is very important to good skin health. We must understand something about our great machine, the body, if we are to take care of it properly. Says Dr. Benjamin S. Frank in his book *No-Aging Diet:* "More people are living longer—thanks to advances in medicine; and more people than ever before are in poor health . . . Loss of energy in the cell is the basic cause of aging and degenerative diseases . . . Since DNA is the cell's blueprint for building new cells, once it is damaged it designs other damaged cells which, in turn, design other damaged ones."

Dr. Frank's recommended diet is, of course, his own, designed to produce the most from nucleic acids, and thought to produce good enzyme stimulation in the body, thereby retarding visible aging. There are diets and there are diets, and many are supposed to do wonders for the complexion and facial muscles.

MILK—DON'T LEAVE HOME WITHOUT (DRINKING) IT

It has become an increasing factor in skin care that diet, a proper and selective one, can play a vital role in maintaining a beautiful skin, and in helping to make middle age a bright and glowing extension of youth rather than a bridge to elderliness. Often people come up with discoveries about nutrition that are worth some attention, whether they are believed by all or just some. Nutritionist Dale Alexander revealed his theory on Michael Jackson's KABC-radio talk show (May 14, 1979) that milk is good not just for the complexion and bones, but for one's sex life as well. He especially praised the effects of raw, certified milk, and of acidophilus milk. He said that his research showed that milk has been of great help to Jewish people in the last few decades.

"Jewish people had for centuries shunned milk with their meals," he said. "I mean Jews of orthodox faith, adhering to all the ancient rites. As a result, varicose veins proliferated among Jewish people. But during the last couple of generations, reformed Jews have been drinking an abundant amount of milk, with or without meals, and the incidence of varicose veins, however hereditary, has diminished greatly and almost disappeared."

Also of significance was a report issued in May of 1979 from the Upjohn Company, in which Dr. William E. M. Lands, professor of biochemistry, University of Michigan at Ann Arbor, states: "We know that all fatty acids can provide metabolic energy by oxidation, and that unsaturated acids can provide fluidity to cellular membranes. As the mechanism of chemically determined control of metabolism is elucidated, it may be possible to construct unsaturated fatty acids synthetically that will offer the maximum nutritive and metabolic value and the minimum deleterious effects when incorporated into a normal diet. Conversely, it may be possible to deliberately impair the metabolism and growth of unwanted cells by adding selected fatty acids to their nutrient pools."

In Chapter VIII, we shall discuss all the vitamins having to do with unsaturated fatty acids. It happens that most people who are concerned with skin conditions want to know what can be done *today* to remedy their conditions, or what to use to cover up the conditions, or to retard such conditions, and what to do to avoid those worry lines, age lines, and skin that insists on looking "tired" when the owner *feels* young and anything but tired.

Whatever aging "cure" anybody introduces, nutrition will be an important part of the remedy. While cosmetics can assuage the outward signs of aging, not too much help can be expected unless we care for ourselves from within. Says Purdue Professor Ronald R. Watson, director of an Indiana study on aging: "Good nutrition and age are inseparably linked. Changes in the diet can prolong life. But changes in the diet depend on how much of a nutrient is eaten, on components of the diet, age when the diet is begun and duration of the diet. We know that processes basic and vital to life can be manipulated and controlled by nutrition."

So maybe we won't have to get those collagen injections, after all.

CHAPTER III

THE SUN—HEALER OR HARMER?

Would that you could meet the sun and the wind with more of your skin and less of your raiment . . .

Kahlil Gibran, *The Prophet*

Among the many causes of lines, wrinkles, and "leathery" skin is our great source of life, warmth, and light—the sun. For all of human history, it has been regarded as the great giver of life, the energizing agent that roams the heavens, ever beaming. But that sun is not to be taken lightly when it comes to its rays. The rays can be harmful to the skin if absorbed in excessive doses, or by persons who are allergic to sunlight.

The skin of all human beings, except albinos, contains at least some dark pigmentation, known as melanin. This pigment absorbs ultraviolet light, like that from the sun's rays. Melanin is responsible for our skin color, just as melanin from melanocytes located in our hair and eyes is responsible for the color of our eyes and hair. Dermatologists say that people with brown and black skin do not have any more melanocytes than people with fairer skin. Differences in skin color, it is explained, depend on how the melanin is distributed in the skin, and on the amount of melanin that the skin is able to produce at one time. The skin of a dark woman carries melanocytes that exude swarms of melanin granules, while the skin of a very fair woman has, from birth, melanocytes pre-programmed to produce only very moderate amounts of melanin. At later stages in life, melanocyte production becomes slower. Darker hair becomes grey. It is said that melanin slows aging.

The skin's ability to absorb ultraviolet light is worth discussing here. When our skin is exposed to sunlight, the melanin-producing melanocyte cells in our bodies suddenly speed up production of melanin, and send large amounts of it to the surface of our skin, like an army of soldiers. Those strong bursts of melanin spread out beneath the filmy surface of the epidermis, creating what is called suntan. Too much sun is surely dangerous if a person's skin is fair. A fair-skinned person may not be able to produce all the melanin that is needed to protect the skin from an excessive amount of sun. Exposure to an excessive amount of ultraviolet rays requires the body to manufacture larger amounts of pigment, and the skin, by its own individual nature and limitations, cannot meet this demand. In some way, this frustrated demand causes the body to release a chemical that swells the blood vessels in the skin. Soreness develops. Fair complexions redden and burn. Another instance of melanin mix-up is sometimes evident in freckled people. Freckles are merely tiny islands of isolated pigment that occur when fragments of active melanocytes become surrounded by groups of less active melanocytes. Some dermatologists call this "mobile melanin." The condition is sometimes evident in fairer women who have exposed their bodies early in life to excessive amounts of direct sunlight. After years of such exposure, any melanin they had begins to deplete. Their melanin is no longer able to rush briskly to the skin's surface to build those protective and beautiful tans. To the horror of these women, their skin becomes crepelike. It begins to collect small brown spots that es-

51

pecially show on the backs of their hands and at breast cleavages.

Some cosmetics manufacturers claim that certain skin-treatment products can remove or cure these conditions. Dermatologists say that the only real help can come from clinical treatment. The drug that has been in use for a long time is tyrosinase, which stimulates production of melanin in sluggish melanocytes. It is also supposed to make "mobile" melanin blend. One of my relatives who underwent tyrosinase injections found that her skin became darker than it had been. She then underwent treatments of phenylalamine, which her doctor told her counterbalanced the darkening effects of the copper component in tyrosinase. After a while, the pools of melanin were no longer visible, and her general skin color returned to normal. Chemosurgery and dermabrasion are sometimes prescribed in severe cases. And some women try to cover these splotches with makeup.

Some people still attest to other remedies for these splotches, often called "liver spots." The manager of one of the largest vitamin centers in Southern California told me that one of the oldest treatments for these spots is castor oil, a nasty-tasting and nasty-smelling medicine that is seldom found in home medicine chests today. It used to be taken as a laxative, but the manager of the store said that he has used it on the splotches on the backs of his hands, and has watched them fade away. Indeed, Dr. D. C. Jarvis, in his 1958 best-selling Fawcett-Crest book, *Folk Medicine,* says this about castor oil: "After success with moles, I became interested in the problem of the brown 'liver spots,' so called, which appear on the face and hands of the aging. I wondered whether they would be favorably influenced by castor oil. I found a patient who had about a dozen such brown spots on the back of each hand and I suggested that castor oil be applied night and morning, rubbing it well into the skin. The patient was glad to try it, for he wanted to get rid of the spots. By the end of one month, they had all disappeared; had I not seen them, I would never have known they had been there."

Recognizing that there was nothing on the market for these "liver spots," the Jeffrey Martin Company of New Jersey came out in 1979 with its Porcelana trade-marked spot-fading cream, at a price of $7.50 for four ounces, and advertised widely on radio and television and in magazines. Its active ingredient is hydroquinone, which for years has been the main substance in skin-bleach creams like Artra, Nadinola, and Black & White. The literature on those products mentions "liver spots," but Porcelana made fading those spots a specialty. But be careful that you don't get it in your eyes. You may be allergic to the hydroquinone.

In Canada, the Philadelphia-based Frances Denney Company's Fade Away has proved a big-selling splotch fader. It also contains hydroquinone.

The Sun, the Leatherizer

Animal skins are left in the sun or under ultraviolet lights for extended periods of time to make them into leather. Human skin is similarly transformed when it is exposed to the sun's ultraviolet rays for extended periods of time. And women who take longer to tan court troubles—lasting ones. Quite often, the results of extended exposure to the sun is leatherized skin. The rays can dry the skin, making it like a prune. That kind of dryness produces hardening and aging in the skin. This can happen even in young women. The sun can quickly destroy skin that would have taken years to age.

Protection for Eye Skin

Just as excessive light from vast blankets of snow can cause one to go snow-blind, sunlight can damage the eyes, too. The sun can also do lasting damage to the delicate skin around the eyes. After years of excessive exposure to the sun, damage to the skin will almost certainly show up sooner or later, usually first as lines around the eyes. On bright, sunny days, we should always keep the eyes and the skin around the eyes protected by a good pair of dark sunglasses. And remember, regular rest will help prevent those shadowy and puffy areas under the eyes. Try sleeping with your head slightly raised on a pillow. This can prevent fluid from collecting in the tissue around the eyes. And as a precaution against the formation of those tiny, dry lines, try using a dab or two of Progrés Eye Creme every night around the area of the eyes.

The Sun Damages Collagen

The sun causes the skin to lose its elasticity by damaging its collagen fibers. As the skin loses its elasticity, the skin fibers in the deeper and supporting layers of the skin, in the dermis, begin to break. This happens more quickly if the skin is also stretched. Collagen damage in the dermis is then reflected in the epidermis, or on the surface. The damage will be more acute if the person is over thirty, even in people with oily skin, which often fends off the effects of the sun better than dry skin does. Oil production generally tends to peak at puberty, and then levels off until menopause. After that, it slowly but steadily decreases in most people with oily skin.

Hormones are rather individual, but their balance is

quite closely related to oil production, and oil production is most often related to a person's metabolism. And so it goes for perspiration, which is often a good sun screen. Among the many women and men who do not perspire easily, some use olive oil as a sun screen as well as a skin-fortifier, especially around the eyes and ears. Olive oil was used as a skin treat even in biblical days.

The Danger of Getting Skin Cancer from the Sun

Excessive exposure to the sun can also harm in another very dangerous way. It can bring on skin cancer. But here again, it has to do with who is by nature more susceptible. Medical people have thought for a long time that our susceptibility to cancer has to do with the melanin we inherit. According to noted cancer specialist Dr. Edmund Klein, associate chief of dermatology at Roswell Park Memorial Institute in Buffalo, New York, eighty percent of the people who get skin cancer are blondes, redheads, and people with blue eyes. In March of 1979, Dr. Klein, who figured in the development of the anti-cancer drug 5-Fluorouracil, described skin cancer to United Press International as an affliction with an "undefinable ethnic factor." As he explained, "Irishmen and Welshmen have a much higher susceptibility toward skin cancer than can be accounted for either by exposure to the sun or by degree of pigmentation." He acknowledged that he has also found numerous cases among blacks and Indians who lacked pigment in some areas of their bodies. He cited "Moon Children" Indians, who live off the coast of Panama. A high percentage of them are albinos, and therefore have a higher than average death rate from sun-caused skin cancer. As a result, they keep out of the sun, and have evolved into a nighttime culture. Skin specialist Klein also cited the darker-skinned people who live around the Mediterranean areas. "The lighter-skinned stock," he said, "was susceptible to sun-caused skin cancer, and died out long ago."

The Sun and the Pill Don't Mix

Clinical tests have found that patches of skin discoloration or pigmentation have been caused by birth-control pills. The sun, according to skin specialists with Clinique Laboratories, "seems to ripen the discoloration." Clinique, one of the nation's major cosmetics firms, advises: "Wear a sun-block product on the brownish area whenever you go into the sun." The Irma Shorell sun line has a Sun Sensitive Sun Creme, which is a completely effective sun block, stopping sunburn, freckling and tanning. It helps prevent blotching and brown spots even from the Pill. Its SPF is 20.

The Browning of America

Men and women all over the world seem to have a desire to be bronze, copper, gold, tan—anything but their inherited color. This desire drives them from their homes and jobs, scattering them into all kinds of prone, supine, and other reclining positions on beaches, rooftops, patios, park lawns, boat decks, and in backyards everywhere. It is often thought that Americans' greatest love affair is with their cars, but it would seem that in summer months and in sunny areas that the love affair is really with the sun. Sixty years ago, no red-blooded ivory-colored American man or woman wanted a tan. For years, such people apologized for reddened or browned faces acquired from prolonged work or other activity in the sun. Even tennis players and golfers used all kinds of head coverings to ward off the sun. Women

56

wore wide-brimmed hats and billowing bonnets to shield their faces from the sun's rays, and did anything else necessary to keep their faces polar white. Men did similar things. People with other than very fair skin indicated that they had been working outdoors, possibly with their hands, rather than indoors, using their minds. Today, looking "tanned and healthy" is a badge of freedom, a sign that the person has been to sunny resorts or on the ski slopes, a sign of being in the bold and boundless class of Clint Eastwood or of the rich New Yorkers who vacation in Florida and Honolulu or on the Riviera.

How the Sun Harms

It takes light rays about eight minutes to race from the sun, ninety-three million miles away, to the surface of your bare body outdoors on Earth. Some of these rays produce visible light, and heat. But the ultraviolet rays, unseen and unfelt, are the bad ones. They do not bounce off your skin, either. They are guaranteed to penetrate all three layers of the skin, something no cosmetic will or can do.

The Damage, Layer by Layer

The skin is the largest organ of the human body. It normally weighs from seven to nine pounds, and is composed of three layers. From the inside out, they are the hypodermis, the dermis, and the epidermis, or outer layer, with which we face the world. Each of the skin's three layers absorbs ultraviolet rays, and reacts differently to them. The rays can and often do pass through all three layers, but each layer has its own ways of blocking or absorbing them. The hypodermis heats up from the rays. The dermis, lying just above the hypodermis and beneath the epidermis, can react with a sore sunburn. The longer ultraviolet rays beat down on the epidermis, and are usually absorbed by it, usually resulting in a suntan. Melanocytes do not immediately send melanin to the surface of the skin to protect it, but the dermis starts them on their way. About three days after strong exposure to the sun, the melanin rises to the surface of the epidermis, in the form of minute granules. They spread out, forming a brownish pigment commonly known as suntan. The ultraviolet rays that radiated through the three layers also have a tendency to darken the melanin that has risen to the skin's surface. In this way, the melanin acts as a sort of sun screen, protecting the skin from further penetration of other ultraviolet rays.

If the bather stays in the sun, the cutaneous, horny layer of the skin thickens and hardens. It won't get any darker, but it does begin to look leathery. On the other hand, a burn rather than a tan is the result when the individual sunbather does not produce enough melanin. And for the successful tanner to keep his or her tan, he or she must keep going back for more sun, making the body produce more melanin in sufficient quantities to replace the granules that are constantly dissipating from the surface of the skin. After all, the outer skin renews itself every twenty-eight days.

Over-Exposure—The Big Danger

The big trouble comes when the sunbather does not discipline him- or herself to stay in the direct sunlight only for a few minutes at a time. He or she can always come back later for more sun. People will lie in the sun all day long, turning over and over again like a hotdog on a spit, getting equally blistered. But can't all that be avoided if one uses a good suntan lotion, you ask? You may also ask, what is a *good* suntan lotion or cream? Or, what is an adequate suntan lotion supposed to do?

A good suntan lotion, or an adequate suntan preparation, serves only one purpose: to screen out a certain percent of the sun's rays, preventing many of them from penetrating the skin. In this way, one *can* tolerate more sun. It permits browning without burning. Such preparations are called sun screens. The ideal sun screen would only be one that could screen out all the harmful rays, permitting only the tanning rays to pass through the layers. Unfortunately, though, some of the burning and tanning rays have virtually the same wavelengths, making it impossible to screen out one without screening out the other. You must select the preparation that you find best for your own skin.

Dermatologist Barbara Gilchrest, who contends that all cosmetics makers should have to prove the efficacy of their treatment products, was asked by an editor of *US* magazine if sun screens were actually any help. Her reply? Absolutely. They seem to be the only products that can preserve the skin, if they are used regularly. And thanks to pressure from the consumer, more and more manufacturers are putting sun screens in moisturizers and makeup.

Some dermatologists contend that almost all signs of lines and wrinkles could be prevented or retarded if people would stay out of the sun. It is probably as impossible to prove such a contention as it is to get people to stay out of the sun. When one looks carefully at the body skin of an elderly person with a lined and wrinkled face, an interesting circumstance becomes evident. The body skin, which has been covered by clothing for most of the person's life, looks years younger, and is free of wrinkles.

With that in mind, I would like some day to study foreign women who keep their faces veiled for religious reasons, to find out if their body skin is smoother than their facial and neck skin.

Prepare for Sunning Beforehand

If you are going to be in the sun for a fairly long time, it is important that you apply a sun screen two or three times. And when you wash or cleanse your skin after the sunbath, do not use strong deodorant soaps. Alcoholic astringents are also out. Use only a very mild soap, with lukewarm water. Then apply a soothing, moisturizing cream or lotion, being careful to rub the solution in by massaging the tissues under the eyes, on and under the chin, and into the areas around the eyebrows, ears, and nose. Massage the temples, neck, and forehead, too. And when you apply the sun screen before sunbathing, always be sure to pat the sun screen into the foregoing areas as well. It is also good to use a sun-screen lotion if you are going to be walking or standing in strong winds, such as those at a parade or during a golf game.

The less distance the rays have to penetrate, the more powerful the rays will be. People who hover around mountaintops during ski meets are never safe, even in winter. Sunlight bouncing off blankets of snow has the effect of a double dose of rays. And the sun packs a greater wallop at noon than it does at four in the afternoon. From about ten in the morning until two in the afternoon, the rays are perpendicular, and they have to slice through less atmosphere than the oblique rays of early morning or late afternoon. In the summer, the sun is more deadly than in the winter, since the sun is closest to the earth in the summer. Don't take the sun lightly on lazy, hazy days of summer, either. It's still up there, sending those rays to Earth, with the same ferocity and capable of doing just as much damage. Smog cuts down the effect of ultraviolet rays, but only slightly.

Many young people throw caution to the winds when they are in the sun, and some of these young people never even heard of any tanning lotion other that those that *help* a person get a tan. In a pamphlet circulated by the Occupational Health Service of the County of Los Angeles, this warning was given to young bathers: "Physicians report that many twenty-year-olds already have sun-damaged skin. The damage is irreversible! Years of overexposure to the sun just adds to the permanent damage. If sun bathing is continued without adequate protection, the twenty-year-olds of today may look like sixty-year-olds when they reach forty. Research recently showed this with studies of human skin samples. Skin from the faces of aging persons was compared with skin from usually covered areas of the same person's body. Facial skin showed pronounced degenerative changes, while body skin retained the elasticity and appearance of the healthy tissue of young skin."

The pamphlet added a precaution against the belief that beach umbrellas can shield the sun's rays. They will shield from sunlight, but not from the rays reflected on your face and body from nearby water and surrounding sand.

Your sun screen should be the kind that will penetrate the epidermis so that the sun screen won't be rubbed off easily by beach towels or washed off when you dip into the water. If you stay in the water for a long time, however, the sun screen will vanish. It should be reapplied when you come out of the water. The sun screen should be nonallergenic, nonirritating, and nontoxic; in other words, completely safe. It should be chemically stable, lasting, and pleasant to use. Avoid lotions that get washed away by perspiration. Also avoid solutions that contain titanium dioxide and zinc oxide. They are too sticky, hard to spread and remove, and may react badly with sun. Sun-screen agents should *always* contain para-amino benzoic acid (PABA).

Teenagers who have treated their acne with retin-A, tretinoin, or vitamin A acid cream or liquid should be aware that the FDA feels that retin-A magnifies the effects of the sun and increases chances of skin cancer. There is no danger, however, if the vitamin A derivative is taken orally. People taking medication (like birth-control pills, Tetracycline, sulfa, diuretics, barbiturates, and/or certain tranquilizers), who have doused with perfumes or after-shave lotions should be especially cautious, as these drugs and/or lotions can cause photosensitizing reactions, *e.g.*, rash or spotting, and can make the skin more susceptible to severe sunburn.

Bonne Bell's Coconut Tanning Butter was ordered off store shelves by the FDA on January 31, 1979, because it contained ingredients that were allegedly irritative to the skin. Some sunbathers prefer Alo-Relief, a good healing tanner. Some prefer Deléal, sold worldwide. Vaseline has its effective Ultra-Vera (Plus UV) sun screen. Any sun screen should contain PABA and vegetable oils. The PABA protects the bather from the ultraviolet rays, and the oils seal in moisture. The oils keep the skin from drying out during the time when the melanin is reacting to the ultraviolet rays.

Lancôme offers a remarkable set of sun lotions marketed under the trade name O de Lancôme pour le Sport, for all skin types and guaranteed to moisturize as they encourage tanning. They filter out the sun's bad rays, and because they are not greasy, they leave the skin feeling soft, smooth, and pliant.

Lancôme's lotion Sun Factor 8, a sun filter, is for use on easy-to-burn areas such as between the breasts, knees, feet, nose, and the back of the neck. It is for sun-sensitive and extra sun-sensitive skin. Sun Factor 6 is a protective tanning lotion, which is meant to be used on the first day in the sun. It is good for sun-sensitive skin, too. Sun Factor 4 is a conditioning tanning lotion for easy-to-tan skin and for sun-sensitive skin, and for the bather who has worn Sun Factor 6 several times in the sun. Sun Factor 4 helps give a deeper tan.

Johnson & Johnson offers Sundown, which boasts lasting powers after a one-time application. It is a PABA derivative that some doctors recommend for sun-sensitive patients. Although it screens out nearly all the sun's harmful rays, the product does permit gradual tanning. Regular water won't wash it away readily, but it comes off easily with soap and water.

Some sunbathers swear by Erno Laszlo's sun oil, because it's greasy, stays on, gives a golden, glistening glow to the skin, and affords very good protection from the sun. Hicks & Greist turn out several suntan lotions and creams, one of which is Alo-Sun. Avon, the world's largest cosmetics company, offers its door-to-door customers an assortment of sun creams and lotions. Pond's (Cheseborough, Inc.) markets many preparations for sunning, some of them under its Vaseline trademark. The Smith, Kline Labs have a popular line of sun lotions that are marketed under their Sea & Skin label. Coppertone is one of the most popular brands on the market, known by sunbathers all over the world. All of these best sellers contain chemical sunscreens.

Another cosmetics manufacturer that offers an all-around regimen of suntan preparations is Germain Monteil. The company's Sun Essentials line was created for sun-loving people of all ages. Each preparation is rich in smoothing moisturizers and is pleasantly scented. The Monteil sun products are marketed in plastic tubes, are easy to carry in a purse, and they appeal to women who not only sunbathe but who do a lot of walking, standing, and sitting in the sun. There are many such people. They sun at pools, on rooftops, in backyards, on apartment verandas, and some of them are often avid spectators at open-air sports events as well. Many of them participate in sports. All of the Sun Essentials contain PABA derivatives, all, that is, except the After Sun Soother. The company markets sun products for all skin types.

Estee Lauder's Outdoor Protective System has a cream specifically formulated for skin protection during sports and other outdoor activities. It is a combination sun block, wind shield, and insulating cream.

The Payot of Paris Health Club for Your Face has in its sun series the Duo Solaire facial tanning cream, in a mirrored compact so that it can be quickly dabbed on in direct sunlight.

The FDA came up with what could be called a PABA grading system, and assigns each sun-screen product a Sun Protection Factor (SPF). The higher the SPF, the more the product protects you from the sun, the longer you can stay in the sun without burning. To deepen a tan, or for an already dark skin, a low SPF sun screen is in order.

Estee Lauder's Outdoor Protective Cream has an SPF of 19. The two-ounce size was introduced at a price of fifteen dollars. The firm markets an After-Sun Lotion, with an SPF of 7, which is a silky lotion that helps keep a suntan if you already have one.

Clinique's Sun Survival line has a Suntan Encourager (SPF 4), which encourages skin that is not overly sun-sensitive to tan without burning, peeling, or blistering. The Sun Block by Clinique (SPF 19) lets you stay in the sun for a longer time. Clinique says that if the product is used regularly, it can help prevent aging caused by the sun. The firm also produces an allergy-tested lip block, a fragrance-free, flavor-free, and invisible shield against sunburn and windburn. It comes in stick form.

Moisturizers should be used before and after sunning, as an all-around precaution, even though many sun products contain moisturizer aids.

With all this in mind, chemists at the Laboratoire Bio-Chemique, in Comedey-Laval, Quebec, came up with a "Take a Tan" pill called Orobronze, which contains a non-toxic coloring agent that brown's the body's fat tissue. The pill's active ingredient is canthexanthine, an FDA-approved ingredient used to color butter and cheese. When ingested, the substance is absorbed in the intestine and stored in the body's fat deposits. It turns the fat tissue beneath the skin brown, and because the skin is translucent, the color shows through as a tan. A box of eighty Orobronze capsules, taken four times a day for fifteen days, sells for under thirty dollars.

For those who do not want to be among the millions who have gotten their tans from within, there are many products on the market that allow you to get a tan from the sun.

Here are some other easily obtained sunning products: Buf Beauty Bar, a moisture-enriched soap, and Apriès le Soleil tan-protecting moisture soap. Both are purportedly good to use before sunning. Buff's Beauty Cream is a good moisture cream to apply after you have been in the sun, as are the Bonne Bell After Sun Moisturizer, Coppertone's Tan Care, and Tropical Blend's After Sun Lotion. Some sun-bathers prefer to use a separate moisture lotion while sunning, although many of the sun screens contain moisturizing ingredients. Finally, it is up to you which name-brand sun product you will use, but always check the label for the Sun Protection Factor—SPF—and judge it according to your own skin type. If you have an olive or brown complexion, or even if your skin is black, select a sun product with a very low SPF—2 to 4; for skin that is average and tans well, try for 4; for a skin that is sun-sensitive, of fairer color and which tans in moderate time, use something with a rating of 6; for the same kind of skin, but with variations from one area to another, stay close to an 8; and for the skin that is very fair, burns quickly, and that seemingly never tans, by all means aim for the higher and highest ratings from 10 to 19. The highest-rated sun screens will let you stay in the sun for hours without any real danger of burning, and if you have any productive melanocytes in your body, they will gradually send what melanin you can muster to the surface, resulting in a beautiful, seductive tan. But play it safe whatever you use. It is probably safer to stay in the sun for only short periods, never for over two hours, and even then only during periods when the sun is not directly overhead. And remember to always keep your skin moist.

PABA Is Your Skin's Best Friend

During a summer trip to Detroit, I chatted with an old friend, a woman who is a vice-president of a very large bank. She told me happily that she was looking forward to vacationing in Acapulco with her family, but that she needed some good advice about the right suntan lotion to guarantee her the deepest tan.

For the first time, I took a good look at her face, at her neck and upper chest, at her arms, at her reddish-blonde hair, and at her sea-blue eyes. Her face, neck, and arms were dotted with thousands of freckles. I asked her if she ever had any trouble tanning.

"Yes," she answered quickly. "I break out in a lot of tiny blisters, just like my father used to do. Somebody told me I should use Eclipse suntan lotion. But I do have trouble getting a tan. But when I come back here from Mexico, I want to show off a golden tan."

I told her that with her freckled condition and

patches of ultra-white skin, she would probably always find it very hard to get a very deep tan, and that she should settle for " a sort of nice pinkish tan."

"That's what I always get," she remarked. "I usually break out in a few blisters before I do, though."

I scribbled out some notes for her, told her to take the sun in small doses, but to go back each day for the same amount of time. Above all, I told her, make sure that any sun products she bought contained PABA.

"What's that?" She looked genuinely puzzled.

I explained the PABA syndrome to her.

I had returned to Los Angeles when my friend returned to Detroit from her vacation in Acapulco. She telephoned me to tell me that the PABA-derivative sun products she had used had helped her get "the prettiest pink-copper tan you'd ever want to see! And my skin did not blister at all. The whole family used it and got a tan."

Just What Is PABA?

It is the common name for para-aminobenzoic acid, and an important factor in the vitamin B complex. It is called a vitamin within a vitamin, in that it occurs in combination with folic acid. It is water-soluble, and is found in yeast, liver, molasses, and wheat germ. It activates intestinal bacteria, stimulating them to produce folic acid, which in turn causes the production of pantothenic acid. Thus, it is a coenzyme, and as such creates a breakdown and body use of health-giving proteins and the formulation of red blood cells. In the tests made thus far, PABA has come through as a shining knight, helping to determine skin health, hair pigmentation, and the health of the digestive system. As a sun screen, it is without a peer, in my opinion.

PABA is manufactured in the body, stored in the

body's tissues, and synthesized by intestinal bacteria. People supplement their own PABA by taking PABA vitamins in doses of up to 100 milligrams, if they are prescribed by doctors for therapeutic purposes. Medical authorities use PABA to treat various skin ailments. It has made grey hair recapture some or most of its original color, and allegedly keeps the restored hair from turning back to grey as long as the person takes daily doses of a combination of folic acid and PABA. And at hospitals all over the world, doctors have attested to the astounding abilities of PABA ointment as a burn healer. This is the same ointment that some skin specialists say can be used to retard skin changes caused by aging, such as dryness, facial lines and wrinkles, and "liver spots."

From dermatology clinics, there are reports that when a PABA treatment is used in cases of lupus erythematosus, a serious skin disorder, the patients show visible signs of improvement. And in the treatment of scleroderma, a disorder that causes the skin to thicken and harden, PABA treatments made the patients' skin gradually become thinner and more pliant and elastic.

Any mega-treatment involving PABA should be undertaken only with the advice and under the attention of a knowledgeable physician, since prolonged ingestion of large doses of PABA can lead to kidney, liver, and heart disorders. And anyone taking sulfa drugs should never ingest PABA tablets or capsules, for the sulfa drugs and the PABA vitamin react very similarly in the body. In fact, back in the 1940s, sulfanilomide was found to have an adverse affect on the sulfanomides in the PABA excretions in the patients' intestinal tracts. Further, scientific research has shown that PABA is so efficient in synthesizing folic acid in the body that when scientists withheld PABA from grey laboratory mice, their hair turned white. The lack of folic acid caused the hair to lose its color.

Adelle Davis points out in her book *Let's Get Well* that our diets should include yogurt, liver, yeast, and wheat germ, if we want to keep our true hair color, adding, "Persons who take five milligrams of folic acid and 300 milligrams of PABA and pantothenic acid daily with some B vitamins from natural sources can usually prevent hair from graying and often restore its color."

The same regimen has been said to produce grand results for people who are losing their hair, and can even make it grow back.

It is a wonder it took cosmetics manufacturers so long to put PABA into their products, especially in suncare products, when as early as the 1940s, medical people had found that PABA worked extremely well to heal burns. The cosmetics manufacturers didn't include PABA until 1969, when scientists at the University of Pennsylvania presented findings to the Society of Cosmetic Chemists, declaring that PABA ostensibly provided very beneficial results in sunburn cases. The story goes that some time thereafter medical scientists in Boston formulated a compound using PABA, which by then was proven to have the ability "to provide protection from sunburn, skin cancer, and aging of the skin."

It would no doubt help many persons seeking the benefits of PABA to pay more than fleeting attention to their diets. It is easy to get PABA through certain foods. In their book on the amazing B vitamins, *Body, Mind and the B Vitamins* (Pinnacle Books, Los Angeles), Ruth Adams and Frank Murray suggest: "The best source of the vitamin PABA is those same foods in which all the other B vitamins are most abundant: meat (especially organ meats like liver), seeds of all kinds and unrefined cereals of all kinds, nuts, leafy green vegetables, brewer's yeast, wheat bran, wheat germ. Be sure to get enough of it."

Caution should never be ignored, however, when one is out seeking a golden tan. Young women should be extremely careful, for reckless abandon can lead, even years later, to a regreted skin condition. An older woman may feel she's gone this far and her skin is like it is, what more harm could come to it? But she should also use intelligence and care, for nothing looks worse than an already lined skin that has suddenly become a leathered, barbecue-brown road map from ultraviolet radiation.

Some Guidelines for Sun Seekers

1. Sunbathe gradually, and only for short periods each day, especially during midday. If you want to stay in the sun for longer periods of time, begin sunning during early morning or late afternoon. Remember that from about 11 A.M. (in summer months) until about 2:30 P.M., the sun's rays are more direct and supercharged with ultraviolet. Besides, it takes repeated sittings in the sun to make the melanin rise to bring out a good tan. It takes from two to three days for the rising melanin to spread out on the epidermis and produce a tan.

2. Most experts agree that five or ten minutes in the morning and five or ten minutes in late afternoon will lead to a good, gradual, painless tan. After three or four days, and after coating your skin all over, you can increase your stay to fifteen minutes or a half hour, but even these stipulated periods should be approached with caution by blondes and redheads, and especially by women with dry skin. Baptizing the epidermis with moisturizers does not preserve the skin. It just cannot cope with sudden, prolonged blasts of sun.

3. Dry skin or not, blonde or brunette, black skin, brown skin, pink skin, or white, a good PABA-fortified sun-screen lotion or cream should *always* be used *first*. Some women do not rub on sun lotions until they have begun to tingle and perspire under the sun. Apply the sun screen *before* you go into the sun, then reapply more as perspiration and water begin to wash it away. In either case, the skin will start out with a protective coating on it. In fact, women who are sightseeing, shopping, gardening, or watching parades or sports events in the sun should apply a light layer of sun screen before leaving home. Watching a tennis or baseball game at high noon under a blazing sun can be an invitation to disaster without a safe sun screen. Your lips, nose, eyelids, cheeks, and chin should get ample applications of makeup made especially for the sun. The Noxell Corporation, manufacturer of the Cover Girl cosmetics, markets an eye shadow that acts as a sun screen and moisturizer.

4. Remember, even after you have safely secured a pleasant suntan, you should use a sun screen before venturing into the sun again. Just because the melanin has spread out on your skin does not mean that the skin has been blessed with a permanent protective shield.

5. After a session in the sun, always cleanse the face and body thoroughly, preferably with a mild facial (not deodorant) soap and lukewarm water. Dry gently with a towel. Then apply a moisturizing cream or lotion, even if your skin is normally oily. Eye creams are a must, for the skin around the eye sockets always gets abused by the sun, and the areas around the eyes don't usually get sufficient moisture. If you cared for your skin before sunning, double the care after.

6. Above all, if you truly care about the condition of your skin, do not forget that the sun is chiefly harmful to any part of the skin that's exposed to it. Sure, sun

rays are warming, whether in the good ole summertime or the mean ole wintertime. The sun is very comforting—for a short time. It invigorates the body at first, but then it tires and debilitates it. It slows the body's pace, and dampens enthusiasm. It explains why people in California move slower than residents of cooler states do. The sun can even cause Meniere's disease and loss of hearing in people who stay bareheaded in the direct sun for too long. The only people sunlight helps are children in their bone-building years, when vitamin D from the sun is needed if they are not getting enough D from foods or vitamin supplements. But all adults should *beware* of the sun. It is definitely harmful. You may think this sounds like an unnecessarily alarmist statement. It is not. The sun can dry you the way it dries clothes on a line. And if you are a fair-skinned person with dry skin, you should be especially careful.

The nastiest thing about that "lucky old sun" is that it does its skin damage in stages. If it doesn't burn you now, it's sure to burn you later. Without protection, your skin will take in the summery sun for several years, and then, right before your eyes, it will begin to crinkle up and "age", no matter how old you are.

Sun sunning cosmetics lines use chemical sunscreens other than PABA, benzophenones, cinnamates, and others long used in Europe only until recently. Deléal's sunscreen is touted (by the company) to be superior to PABA. But take your pick, remembering that any sunscreen is better than none.

CHAPTER IV

BAN-LINES, CLAIMS
AND DISCLAIMERS

Time has touch'd me gently in his race,
And left no odious furrows in my face.
Crabbe, Tales of the Hall

Dermatologists, who are normally concerned with skin diseases, often hasten to warn cosmetics users to be careful with advertised creams and lotions and suggest that indiscriminate use may lead to skin disorders worse than those thought to be causing their original condition. Indeed, to most medical people, any skin condition is medical, not cosmetic, but can you imagine what it would be like if most women went to dermatologists rather than to cosmetics consultants? True, in the past, cosmetics makers were thought to be solely makers of facial paints, but time and the public demand changed all that. It is also true that ever too frequently some company does turn out some kind of product that it vaguely claims will *cure* certain skin conditions. In fact, some advertisers come mighty close to saying that their products will *remove* kinks in skin, lines in skin, and wrinkles in skin. Some are honest enough to say their lotions and creams do that only *temporarily.* And for most women with lines and wrinkles, just getting temporary relief is a godsend, even if the results last for only a few hours. But when they are at home, looking in the mirror at the less noticeable conditions on their faces, they begin to crave something more permanent that will remove or suppress these conditions.

The answer appears to be more and more that help for lines and wrinkles caused by aging and/or skin abuse can and must come from a studied and practiced regimen of all-around body, dietary, mind, and cosmetic grooming. If riding a bike can stimulate blood circulation in the legs, surely other exercises can stimulate renewed circulation in the upper torso, neck, and face.

Daily facial and neck massages surely help tired skin to come alive and flourish. Surely, appropriate vitamins and the right diet can nourish skin cells. Surely, a happier frame of mind can erase depressed looks on gloomy faces. Surely, abstinence from excessive amounts of liquor and cigarettes can help the body produce a healthier condition that is bound to show on the face. And surely, a good skin-care regimen, practiced faithfully each day, and combined with the right cosmetics, can help complement the benefits sure to be derived from the foregoing.

I would never suggest that all women can get along without cosmetics, no matter how well they take care of themselves. There are times, when everybody has to use something on the skin. Oh, yes, some "beauty experts" urge a *natural* approach to beauty and suggest that skin beauty is fully attainable "without fads and dangerous cosmetics." First, all cosmetics are not dangerous. Lecithin, cider vinegar, B-6, and kelp may be excellent for a Mary Ann Crenshaw, but may not be a savior for *your* unique body. In some people, but not all, lecithin can help the skin become soft and supple. And a treatment within needs a treatment without. Even dermatologists prescribe ointments. Some women with extremely dry and cracking skin could eat lecithin by the quart daily and still require moisturizers to help their condition.

Some women are so afraid of "dangerous" cosmetics that they carry around little nitrazine-paper kits in their purses, testing cosmetics like female Sherlock Holmes, ever seeking 4.5 acid level. They have been told that the normal acidity of the skin is "somewhere around 4.5," varying somewhat according to the oiliness of the tester's skin. So they go to a drugstore, buy a small packet of corn-colored nitrazine papers, pegged at 4.5. Then they dip a slip of that nitrazine paper into a cream or lotion to see if the product is highly alkaline and possibly subject to upsetting the acid balance, or acid "mantle," of their skin. If the nitrazine paper turns blue, the woman is wary of the product. It is strongly alkaline and probably dangerous. If the paper turns purple, the woman hurries out of the store, leaving the product out of sight and out of mind.

Almost everyone's pH factor is different. A skin with a 5.0 pH factor is close to perfection. The pH level of most shampoos is 5.0 or higher, indicating they are good for the average and normal skin. Anything under 4.8 is not very good for the skin. The acid level of most good skin varies from about 4.8 to 5.7. The acid level of one cream may be good for one woman but not for another.

If she does not know her own skin's acid balance, a woman can stick those little papers into every cream jar in a store and still not know if the cream is the absolutely right one for her. And if she is going to be exact, she needs to buy specialized cosmetics only, or have her acid balance checked by a dermatologist and then have an Eddie Senz-like firm prepare a product keyed to her exact acid balance. The truth is, most cosmetics are suitable for average skin, and a woman whose skin has already begun to show lines and wrinkles is in no position to run around being a stickler for acid balance. She is already "out of balance." Too much sun, too much booze, too much smoking, too little attention to her skin, and possible hereditary factors have already shot her pH factor and acid mantle collectively to hell. Almost any good skin-cleansing, skin-toning, and skin-treatment cosmetic line will help.

A True Story

I recall one day when an elderly lady walked up to me in the I. Magnin department store in Pasadena and asked me what she could buy to make her look nice for dinner that evening. She added that she had tried to apply adequate makeup before she left home but had been unable to accomplish the job to her satisfaction. I looked into her face. There were no fine lines. There were real lines. They had been with her a long time. There were wrinkles. I had her sit down, beamed a soft light on her, and made sure her facial skin was clean. I ascertained its texture in all areas, applied a light moisturizer with quick-penetration qualities, and then left her for a few minutes, while plumping action set in and her face took on a glowing firmness. In applying the moisturizer, I made sure to press into her skin hard enough to stimulate the blood flow and to spring the skin to life. She began to look more alive. Then I noticed small brown spots that had been hiding between the lines before I applied the moisturizer. I used a sure-fire flaw concealer on them, let it dry, and watched the flaws disappear. Then I applied selective makeup. Not only did she look more beautiful to me, she looked like a new woman to herself. Off she went to her dinner date, happy as a lark. The next day, she was back, beaming, thanking me for doing what was routine for me, but what was special for her. I wrote down for her the steps I had taken and why, and the name of each cosmetic item I used on her face. I also gave her, as briefly as possible, a daily regimen to follow—skin care, diet, vitamins, and exercises. True, she bought cosmetics, but she would now feel more assured and knowledgeable using them. Her whole system was on the road to improvement. Would her lines go away? Some of them would, if she followed the routine. The remaining ones would add to her dignified look. At least her face would no longer look tired. She had achieved both an inner glow and an outer glow.

Facial Transformations Are Not Easy

The job of transforming a tired face into an untired one is not easy. Most women wait until the first wrinkle turns into many before taking action. The skin always requires a nutritious diet, proper cleansing, moisturizing, lubrication, protection from the sun, fresh air, exercise, and relaxation. So many people take better care of their feet than they do their faces. True, some women, and even men, feel that to give regular attention to their faces is indulging in a form of narcissism. Far from it. Beautiful skin requires dedication, daily dedication. A properly cared-for face will generate much of its own color, negating the need for much makeup, except for some eye shadow. And clean, clean, clean. Keep it clean. Whether you prefer special soaps and water or manufactured cleansers, do keep the skin clean.

Deep cleansing removes dirt and grit particles and pollutants without removing natural skin oils. There are products that get rid of excess natural oil on the skin, but it takes a few days for these excess oils to disappear. Cleansers should be applied to the face and neck with a firm, determined massaging action. Always rinse with lukewarm water. Cleansers often miss some of the impurities you want to remove from your face and neck. That is when toning is in order. A good toner removes this grime, and also whisks away dead surface-skin cells, tightens up the skin pores, and texturizes the skin. A moisturizer can then replenish necessary moisture. Some moisturizers retain moisture, forming a barrier against moisture loss, even bringing in new moisture from the air. In some climates, this is highly important, for we often go from outdoors to inside, into temperatures that are immediately detected by the skin and to which the skin instantly reacts. Overly warm rooms can cause makeup-disturbing perspiration. Overly cold rooms can cause the skin to shrink, resulting in a sudden pasty look.

There are so many cosmetics lines on the market that any woman can find the one right for her, if she knows what to look for. There are skin treatments to stave off wrinkles and those for coping with wrinkles that have already arrived. Coty, Mary Quant, Almay, Aida Grey, Faberge, Doak, Charles Revson, and Max Factor are among the most well-known that have their own specialized products for cleansing, toning, moisturizing, firming, and replenishing the skin.

Skin-care products today are directed at the woman who is over twenty-five. Cover Girl and Oil of Olay hit hard at the over-twenty-five set. But some of the skin-care advertising affects the under-twenty-five women, too, prompting them to begin caring for their skin while they are still young. It's possible that it won't be too long before lines and wrinkles will be as hard to find as varicose veins.

Alexandre de Markoff brought out a Lotion for Lines, two oz. for around twelve dollars, a good under-makeup lotion that removes facial lines. And for less money, a three-month supply for five dollars, Walgreen customers were able to buy Secret Miracle, also a temporary wrinkle smoother, which was supposed to banish wrinkles for eight full hours—an average working woman's day. But the one lotion that captured the attention of millions was Jovan's Wrinkles Away, five oz. for under eight dollars, another temporary wrinkle wonder smoother, which goes to work in five minutes and transforms lines and wrinkles into smoothness for "a good part of the day or night." Wrinkles Away hit the mass market with a big bang, and sales of it are still ringing on cash registers everywhere. It is also a single-remedy product that does not require the co-use of other supplementary products. In fact, the smoothers should all be regarded as makeup rather than as treatment products, since their benefits are basically temporary. Proper treatment can cause long-term benefits and changes, unlike makeup, which is kept on for a while and removed later. Using wrinkle lotions is not at all like putting on makeup, which can be removed later by cold cream or Albolene cream.

With all their temporary qualities, some of the wrinkle removers are harsh when they come in contact with skin, since some of them are primarily made of albumin, or egg white. I would not recommend long-term use of any of them. The skin may get tired of being "propped up" all the time, as if by a crutch, and pretty soon will rebel by remaining saggy, no matter how much temporary wrinkle lotion is applied to it. In fact, such steady diets of momentary correction might make the lines and wrinkles much more pronounced and even unsightly. These lotions allow the skin to do things it would not naturally do. In time, if no other substances are used, the skin may refuse to react.

Revlon's Etherea line offers day and night products for skin tending toward lines and wrinkles. Its Humistat is an instantly absorbed, all-day emollient lotion that adds and attracts moisture. And it leaves no visible residue. A drop spreads swiftly and smoothly. It vanishes. Humistat's penetration performs without undue rubbing or skin stretching. Etherea does not recommend pressure massaging. Some women say that Humistat makes their skin appear to need no makeup at all. Added makeup does not build up in the lined areas, and no orangy tint appears later in the day, even if there are temperature changes. Humistat, one oz. for around eighteen dollars, contains propylene glycol—a combination of glycerine and alcohol—as one of its active ingredients. Propylene glycol absorbs moisture and is a proven wetting agent.

Etherea's oil-rich Guardian, one oz. for around thirteen dollars, is a nighttime emollient and neither adds nor attracts moisture. Guardian is exactly what its name implies. It develops a barrier that prevents moisture loss, and is normally applied after the application of Humistat. Like Humistat, Guardian vanishes immediately after it is applied, leaving no greasy look or pillow stains. Etherea boasts that "Guardian just leaves you looking younger and smoother than you did an instant before."

Halston provides skin-treatment products for all skin types, and advises that a specific regimen be used prior to the application of makeup. Halston markets a skin cleanser that is lightweight and non-drying, and that helps soften the skin while it washes away makeup, dirt, grit, and excess natural oils. It can be rinsed or tissued away. The Halston Toner, a non-alkaline product enriched with humectants, a substance widely used in creams and lotions to preserve moisture, is recommended as a follow-up item. One of the earliest humectants known was a combination of rose water and glycerine, used even now as a hand lotion. Its ability to preserve moisture is a known fact. Humectants often used in skin emollients are glycol, glycerine, sorbital, and propylene. Halston's eye cream, which contains propylene glycol, glyceryl, rice bran oil, camelia oil, sorbitan, and collagen, has also been praised. It is best used sparingly at night, after toning and before applying Halston's Moisturizer.

Helena Rubinstein, which markets the milk-protein Skin Dew moisturizing emulsion for dry skin, highlights the importance of its Existence Accelerated Action Cream which is imported from France, and sells at forty-five dollars for two ounces. It heats up the skin, and stimulates circulation. It contains DNA, and is a good firmer. With its remarkable stimulating abilities, it is fine for use on the throat, where there is often not enough stimulated circulation. Of it, the company says, "Use this precious imported cream sparingly, stroking upward over cleansed face and throat until cream melts into skin. Use Existence as your regular night cream, or alternate every two weeks with Helena Rubinstein's Skin Life Cream." Existence sometimes stimulates irritation and a rash. But even the best throat creams may cause some irritation.

The Princess Marcella Borghese Company has perfected a five-step skin-care system that does "more for your complexion than any single cream or lotion you can buy." The line is called Catalyste, and consists of a carefully conceived regimen of five hormone-free products: (1) Cleansing Sequence Cream, (2) Equalizing Sequence Lotion, (3) Day Sequence Lotion, (4) Night Sequence Cream, and (5) Synergistic Sequence Intensifying Oil, which, when used during the skin's normal twenty-eight-day renewal cycle, should do wonders for facial skin. Borghese claims that the sequential products worked wonders in clinical tests on women in Cannes, Lausanne, Copenhagen, and Vienna. Borghese forbids the use of any other facial cosmetic while the Catalyste program is being used. Emphasis is on the synergistic effect, the total effect of the interrelated action of all the components, which thereby enhances the effect of each independent component.

It may seem at times that you need a college education to decipher clearly some cosmetics companies' claims. The woman consumer wants something to rectify an unwanted facial condition. She knows what she wants *off* her face, and a zillion cosmetics firms are always telling her, in profuse and nebulous words, what she should put *on* her face. To be sure, it is an easy thing for any person to grab a household dictionary and get a definition of an unfamiliar word encountered in a high-flown cosmetics ad. But when those ads are full of hints, intimations, ploys, and suggestions, while being vague, please be careful. If you don't know what you're doing, ask somebody. If you don't know what a product is supposed to do for you, forget it, no matter how enticing and fascinating the advertisements sound.

Imaginative cosmetics copywriters are experts at creating the *impression* that a certain cosmetic will do what a buyer *hopes* it will do. *Penetrate* and *absorb* are probably two of the most misused and misleading words from the cosmetics copywriter's lexicon. Some companies create and sell the impression that a woman can raise her own nutrient garden in the potting soil of her skin, absorbing proteins, vitamins, and all sorts of other nutrient goodies for "undernourished skin cells" just by slathering on this or that cream or lotion. If these concoctions could do as much for the skin as they can for the user's mind, they would truly be doing a lot of good. Unfortunately, that is not always the case. The woman who gets live-cell injections under controlled conditions is sure to get benefits never to be obtained by the woman who merely rubs a live-cell substance on her skin.

Contrary to popular belief, it *is* possible to introduce

proteins and vitamins into the body through the skin. Scientists have been successful in doing this, but it has become something of a lay practice as well. Various skin-care cosmetics now contain ingredients that can be absorbed through the skin; however, they do not always produce instant benefits. That is why the makers of these products tell you that you must keep on using them for a given length of time before you can expect to see and feel the desired results. After all, bad skin conditions do not develop overnight, either. Skin-treatment products that require steady and controlled use, along with supplemental products and exercises, will more likely lead to lasting results than a bottled wonder that purportedly gives you heavenly beauty and perfect skin in five minutes. It's easy to fool somebody who wants to be fooled, and it is difficult to get a woman to stay on a strict regimen unless she has been frightened half to death by a new wrinkle.

Top-line cosmetics makers work their strategists and chemists overtime figuring ways to add various skin nutrients to their products, and whenever possible, they add the nutrients and advertise them. They are permitted to do so by the FDA, the Food and Drug Administration, the federal agency that periodically tests cosmetics products not only to see if they do what they claim, but to see if they are safe. That is why every so often the FDA issues a warning against the use of some ingredient found in a cosmetic product.

In April of 1979, the FDA urged the cosmetics industry to remove from its products any ingredient that could combine with other chemicals to form potentially cancer-causing nitrosamines. It happened that the American Chemical Society's researchers at the Thermo Electron Research Center in Waltham, Massachusetts, and the Massachusetts Institute of Technology (MIT) had issued a report saying they had found a

83

cancer-causing agent, or a combination of agents, in such cosmetics items as skin lotions and shampoos. Their report claimed that they had found very small amounts of a nitrosamine called N-nitro-societhanolamine (NDELA) in certain skin lotions, and that they had concluded that the nitrosamine was possibly formed by a reaction between nitrate and another additive during the preparation of the products. Medical researchers had some time before found that NDELA can cause liver cancer in rats. The Massachusetts researchers said they feared that some of the NDELA in the skin lotions could be absorbed by the skin. The FDA checked out the Massachusetts report, and issued a warning to the cosmetics industry.

As I have already pointed out, nearly any ingredient can cause irritation or other harm to the body if it is mixed in unsafe proportions or combines with certain ingredients. Some of the world's deadliest poisons are used to cure diseases. But there is always a grave danger in using some cosmetic that does not cause instant irritation and rashes but that sets carcinogens into motion. That is why several years ago the FDA ordered that a certain ingredient be removed from skin-bleach creams. The ingredient could be absorbed into the body through the skin and cause brain damage. It is amazing that so many women who will carefully count calories will eagerly apply any beauty item without examining it. Skin potions containing hormones such as estrogen are also frowned on by the FDA.

Help from Yesterday

Remedies for lines and wrinkles are not found only in recent cosmetics products. The recent ones seem glamorous, even if they cost more. But there are cosmetic remedies that have been with us for years, although they are not universally known because they were never promoted with gigantic advertising budgets.

Cocoa butter is still with us, after generations of use by sunbathers and people trying to soften their skin after exposure to cold weather. These people must find the results satisfying, for cocoa butter is still used all over the world. Hand creams often contain cocoa butter. Babies' bottoms are alternately hand-painted with Johnson's baby oil and with cocoa butter. And mothers' stretch marks are still being faded by cocoa butter.

And never let us forget castor oil. Just as I told you earlier that castor oil is a time-tested remedy for those brown "liver spots" on the backs of aging hands, so, too, castor oil is good for rubbing away wrinkles. I say "rubbing away," for a good deal of the treatment comes not from just the application to the skin of the cocoa butter or castor oil, but from the brisk and determined massaging of the hands and fingertips. Rub it in. Rub, rub, rub determinedly. You surely can't hurt those lines and wrinkles. If anything, you will awaken the dormant skin cells, cause the blood in them to flow more freely, and aid the skin-softening action of the oils. I know you will look at your skin immediately after one of these ritualistic treatments, to see if anything has happened to the lined areas or wrinkled surfaces. Do not panic. Persevere. Those unwanted skin conditions took years of neglect and abuse to develop, while you were looking and did not see. There is help all around you—skin-care lotions and creams, masks, packs, facial exercises, foods, and vitamins. Just think, if vitamin A can remove a pimple virtually overnight, it surely can do wonderful things for you if you ingest a proper amount of it daily. Vitamin A and vitamin E, when rubbed into lines and wrinkles, can help eradicate the condition.

While on the subject of help from yesterday, I know one woman in her sixties who swears by garlic as a skin aid. Almost before my eyes, her acutely lined facial and neck skin and the dry and puffy skin around her eyes improved, leaving her with a glow and vigor she had probably experienced only during her youth. How did she do it? She told me she had followed the advice of one of her relatives from the "old country" and had gone on a "garlic diet," sprinkling the stuff into her food and taking garlic tablets daily, drinking lots of water, exercising her body and facial skin, and getting lots of rest. Even her hair had begun to grow abundantly. Her loose and saggy skin had become healthfully taut and firm. Her whole attitude had changed. She glowed all over.

Later, I checked on the nutrient content of garlic and learned that the odorous little root is an ace digestive, circulatory, and blood regulator, as well as a source of minerals, vitamins, enzymes, calcium, oxygen, iron, and other elements that body tissues need to be healthful. But, as John Lust states in *The Herb Book* (Benedict Lust Publications, 1974): "The problem with garlic is that when you use it you inherit the smell along with the benefits."

The Great Feminine Fear of Water

It is astounding how many women act as if they secretly fear regular drinking water. Of course, the public drinking water in some areas does leave a lot to be desired. But in those places, one can always buy bottled purified, mineral, or spring water. Wise when you consider how many women actually buy the rather costly aerosol containers of water imported from France and tapped from elsewhere just to spray on their faces for cleansing and cooling. A lot of medical people never cease to be astounded at the many women who "accidentally on purpose" hold off drinking plain water until they finally come down with a liver, kidney, or bladder ailment and their faces become as arid as the Sahara. Maybe nobody ever told them that water is the body's most abundant nutrient, that it accounts for roughly two-thirds of the body's weight, and it plays a dominant role in digestion, circulation, absorption, and excretion.

Water is the chief transporting vehicle for nutrients flowing through our bodies and is vital for all bodily functions. Can you imagine a person using all kinds of moisturizing lotions and creams and at the same time neglecting to drink enough water daily to keep the inner tissues functioning properly? That is exactly what happens in women and men by the hundreds of thousands. They may even disdain or shun eating fruits regularly, not knowing that fruits and vegetables are an excellent source of pure water—one hundred percent oxygen and pure hydrogen.

Some women never perspire, and wonder why.

Older persons generally evaporate about a quart of water a day, in contrast to an adult desert dweller, who experiences a daily water loss of up to ten quarts. In either case, the body contains approximately forty-five quarts of water. On the average, through excretion and perspiration, a person loses about three quarts of water each day.

Understanding Your Skin Conditions

Some people do not have the faintest idea how the mind and body work together to benefit or harm us. Many of us buy the latest in skin-care cosmetics to "treat" worried-looking faces, and yet do nothing to temper the possible causes of the condition. We actually add insult to injury by assaulting ourselves with constant worry and constant liquor, coffee, sugared drinks, and nicotine. Not only will the skin fail to survive under such conditions, but it is probably too much to expect that the body will survive, either. We must try to understand the relations and co-relations of skin-care cosmetics, exercise, and good nutrition, and the actions of certain vitamins not only on our skin, but in our bodies, where they work to nurture our skin from within. If a daily ingestion of RNA/DNA 100 mg tablets can do wonders to clear up facial pimples and make one feel new vigor, it must be because the tablets are supplying something the body was not getting in the first place. If lecithin taken orally can help moisturize body tissues, it should also follow that skin-care cosmetics containing lecithin should help moisturize the skin as well.

Some skin experts say that whatever is used as an emollient around the eyes should be accompanied by regular exercises. One cosmetic giant, Lancôme, maker of the Progrés Eye Creme, says: "Never pull, rub or stretch skin around the eyes." Payot says that the eye areas should get daily but gentle fingertip massages. Dr. M. J. (Joe) Saffon, known for the "Hollywood Instant Face Lift" technique, says that areas around the eyes are the only part of the face that will not respond to exercises. Dr. J. Frank Hurdle, author of *The Common Sense Health Manual,* contends that the area around the eyes should get rubbed and massaged. Personally, I feel that the area around the eyes benefit from gentle massaging. The application of eye creams and eye packs helps, too. This area also gets stimulation from the applying and removal of cleansers. The skin may be delicate, but it's been with us for a long time. Some eye creams with vitamin A soothe and lubricate the area around the eyes as well.

Sleep is also vital. What good is an eye cream for puffy eyes with dark circles under them, especially when the condition was caused by a lack of rest, or liquor, or inadequate diet? Conditions caused by those things cannot be helped significantly by massage, either. And I never liked the skin-peeling ritual for the areas around the eyes. Really, skin trouble around the eyes indicates that the trouble is more than skin deep.

You can rub cocoa butter or castor oil into your skin daily to soften and lubricate it. Or, if you have decided on a good line of cosmetic products offering these same skin-softening and lubricating benefits, you can use them instead. If your own cosmetic product is moisturizing enough, use it. I shall not tell you to make a cosmetics factory in your home, dipping from a helter-skelter assortment of natural herbs, oils, vitamins, roots, proteins, and the like, measuring them, cooking and refrigerating them, and all that. It's too much for the average woman, unless she has nothing else to do each day but to collect cosmetics ingredients, mix them, prepare creams and lotions, and apply them. Even a pharmacist doesn't have that kind of time. But when you know what your skin is like, what it needs, where to find it, and what sort of regimen to follow, you can dedicate yourself to a regimen that will not interfere with your everyday life, and you can happily watch as changes take place in your skin. Watch your own skin regenerate, and be happy with the changes. If you know what you want to change, you can make every effort to change it.

PRESERVATIVES AND "NATURAL" COSMETICS

There are some beauty "experts" who are sold completely on their own "natural" formulas for skin health, and who condemn all cosmetics because they contain preservatives. Well, almost everything today contains preservatives, if it is expected to last for more than a day. Virtually every food contains preservatives, for most of us cannot walk around picking our fruits from trees and vegetables from the ground. It would be good if we could get most of our foods from the fresh-produce counters of the best stores, but there are times when we resort to canned items, and they all have preservatives. A preservative is used in cosmetics to provide protection against contamination. Preservatives prevent decomposition due to microbial multiplication. Water, lanolin, and cocoa butter are excellent breeding grounds for germs. And we have a habit of leaving jars and bottles uncapped, thereby making it possible for the ingredients to pick up more germs. Just as humectants keep cosmetics from drying out, preservatives keep cosmetics from becoming sitting germ traps. According to Ruth Winter in her *Consumer's Dictionary of Cosmetic Ingredients*, "A cosmetic preservative should be active at low concentration against a wide range of microorganisms, and over a wide acidity/alkalinity range." According to cosmetic chemists, it must also be compatible with the other ingredients, be non-toxic, non-irritating, and nonsensitizing. It also should be colorless, odorless, and stable, as well as inexpensive and easily incorporated into the product. Quaternary ammonium compounds, such as benzalkonium chloride, are widely used preservatives. So are the various alcohols such as ethyl and isopropyl. Aldehydes, particularly formaldehyde and benzaldehyde, are common preservatives, as are the phenolic compounds, such as phenol and p-chloro-m-cresol. Essential oils, such as citrus and menthol, have been used for hundreds of years as preservatives. Essential oils also are used to preserve the fatty products in cosmetic creams and lotions. Such substances are called antioxidants. They prevent the production of unpleasant colors and odors. Examples of such antioxidants are benzoic acid and

BHA. BHA (butylated hydroxyanisole), which is insoluble in water, can, like other preservatives, cause allergic reactions in some persons.

Acid Versus Alkali

Acid mantles, acid balance, pH factors, and such are topics for heated discussion among many anti-cosmetics spokespersons. A technical definition of the pH factor is given here by Ms. Winter: "The degree of acidity or alkalinity (known as the pH) of a product is important in cosmetics because too little or too much of either may irritate the skin. Furthermore, the formulation of a product is dependent upon properly maintaining the intended pH. Citric acid, widely used as the acid, and ammonium carbonate, an alkali, are frequently found in cosmetic formulations. Buffers and neutralizing agents are chemicals added to cosmetic formulas to control acidity or alkalinity in the same way that acids and alkalies might be added directly. Some common chemicals in this class are ammonium bicarbonate, calcium carbonate, and tartaric acid."

The problem is that women have become fearful about the pH factor. As we have already noted, the pH factor is the degree of acidity or alkalinity of any solution, whether it is a soap or a cosmetic. Soaps are not cosmetics, although one might think they are the way they are so often grouped together with cosmetics. For a time, hardly a cosmetics firm promoted soap. In fact, they urged the use of cosmetic cleansers instead. Only the Procter & Gamble and Lever Brothers people promoted the cleansing power of soaps. But if hair shampoos (liquid soaps) must carry pH factors, one would think that cakes and bars of facial soaps would be marked also. And they are. A pH of 7 is neutral; under 7 is acid, and over 7 is alkaline. Soaps are the least likely to pass a 4.5 or 4.8 to 5.7 pH test. After all, they are not cosmetics anyway. A soap with a pH factor over 7 no doubt is a detergent or strong deodorant soap, and may remove the skin's natural protection right along with surface dirt and grit. This natural protection is a natural germ barrier, and when it is erased germs rush in. When that natural barrier is removed, the condition is instantly set up for the eruption of blackheads and acne. Caution should be used with soaps, even with those that are supposed to contain cold cream, for they can have some mighty high pH factors.

Only recently has the public become aware of pH factors, acid mantles, and acid balances. For years, the only cosmetics companies emphasizing pH factors were Erno Lazslo and the RedKen people, the latter spurred by the pH theories of Jheri Redding, now the main force behind the beauty-shop-promoted Jhirmack products, which we shall examine later on in this chapter. Those other cosmetics firms, who made sure all along that their products met normal pH requirements, probably will be concentrating more and more now on convincing their consumers of the pH factors in their products.

Women who have not used soaps and water for facial cleansing may not know which soaps are mild enough for them. It is worth noting that numerous top-line cosmetics makers have added mild face soaps with low pH factors to their facial-treatment lines. You should look for a soap with a pH of about 3 or 4, with a maximum of 5. No more. Lather first on the hands, and the apply the *lather* to the face, the way you would apply a cream. Rinse thoroughly, almost ritualisticly, dousing the face from twenty to thirty times, letting the water act as a massaging vehicle. I know one woman who uses a gentle-set Water-Pik as a Jacuzzi-like spray massage for her face after using Germain Monteil's Clarity

Super Soap lather on it. The soap cleanses and refreshes, but she says she gets a tingle from the water spray that beats the tingle cosmetic cleansers are advertised to give.

Age Is Not a Sure Barometer

In order to keep lines and wrinkles under control, we should never forget or ignore the value of certain ingested vitamins. Although I shall take up the topic of vitamins later, I must emphasize the importance of B vitamins, and especially B-2, or the riboflavin vitamin. A deficiency in B-2 leads to lines anywhere, on anybody. We should not get into the habit of believing that lines and wrinkles have to do specifically with aging. A number of factors can cause the onset of wrinkles, including heredity. I have seen women afflicted with various illnesses who at age fifty, sixty, and seventy had no signs of lines or wrinkles in their faces. They were plump women. Few fat women get facial lines. I know several fifty-six-to-sixty-year-old women who were told to lose weight because of diabetic conditions. After they shed the weight, their faces began to develop deep lines. Where there was once plump, elastic tissue, the flesh had shrunk, giving way to deep valleys and wrinkles. After some time in which they observed good dietary habits and proper facial care, their reduced facial skin had a new firmness and suppleness, and the lines had vanished. Age did not have anything to do with these conditions and changes.

I saw in a national magazine photos, side by side, of baseball managers Sparky Anderson and Billy Martin. The deep lines in their faces instantly caught my attention, and made me wonder. Neither man was "aged." Anderson's age was listed as forty-five, and Martin's as fifty-one. Worry lines? Alcohol? Heredity? Maybe, I thought, a combination of all three and then some. But those lines were probably mainly caused by the fact that both men spent a major portion of their lives in the sun on baseball fields. I was willing to bet that the backs of their necks, always exposed to the sun, were roughened and reddened from those years of exposure.

I know a woman of fifty who has been one of my best cosmetics customers. When she first came to me, her face had numerous lines that had begun to form, she told me, when she was thirty. She has lost most of those lines now, but when I first saw her she was a humdinger. She told me she had spent much of her younger life in the open air, swimming, playing tennis, skiing, in the sun all the time. Recently, she introduced me to her mother. I saw the resemblance at once. But whereas the daughter, at fifty, had an angular, more bony face, the mother, at seventy, still had a full, rounded, plumpish face—and not a single line or wrinkle anywhere. The mother was proud of her face, and quickly boasted that she had never had a face lift. She confessed that she had not used many facial creams and lotions, either.

"I started taking care of my skin when I was fifteen," this vigorous, beautiful and youthful-looking woman of seventy told me. "And even before then, when I was a small child back in Niagara Falls, New York, my mother taught me that rosy cheeks in the snow were a pretty thing, but that cold weather would harm my face. When I went out to play in the snow, she would have my face filmed with cold cream, which she'd remove when I was back in the house. And I kept out of the direct sun for years. I figured that if God wanted me to be brown, he would have had me born with brown skin. At times, I use cold cream as a pore cleanser, but most of the time I have used a mild Sayman's soap, a warm water rinse, a cold water sealer, and a towel. I use cosmetics, but very lightly, and I never use any pasty eye shadow on the soft skin around my eyes. I have always been particular about my diet and vitamins, and I exercise my facial muscles all the time."

Truly, a walking case history of a woman with beautiful facial skin. Apparently, age had no harmful effects.

Furthermore, the woman said she did not need eyeglasses to read. Her vitamin intake probably gave her enough A and B-2 (riboflavin) vitamins, assuring less eye trouble. Vitamin B-2 also prevents wrinkling, by retarding those "premature" signs of aging.

So much cosmetics advertising stresses the need to be on guard against premature aging, which begins at about the age of forty-five, according to many of the ads. Women are frightened that their skin will begin to look like a "dried prune" by that age if they don't use this or that product. They are told that appearance of lines and wrinkles represents "premature aging signs." Really? Should aging necessarily be equated with lines in the face? It cannot be repeated too often; no single cosmetic item or multi-item line alone can remove those socalled aging signs. They can help, if they are the right items and used properly and long enough. Miracles do happen, if you wait long enough. But in these cases, your body itself needs to help. DNA enzyme factors, however hereditary, should never be discounted. Just imagine that some scientist suddenly discovered an eternal youth drug that was to be injected into your body, and that you were told that this drug would prevent your face from aging. Now suppose that you were afraid to get the injection, but that you would have the same mixture applied in cream form to your face. After all, that's where the trouble is, you say. That's where it's showing. So you apply it on your face rather than ingesting it. You would have to wait and watch a long, long time for those desired results to show. What if the

95

concoction were absorbed through the skin? It still could not make the skin act on its own, totally independent of DNA-directed cellular action that works upon the body as a whole. The face and neck are not separate from the rest of your body. In order to make changes on the outside, some kind of change has to be taking place on the inside, too. Constant mental stress will offset whatever benefits are to be gained. Stress, at any age, is sure to add lines. You may take a boatload of stress, or anti-stress, vitamins, or a ton of the Valium-like tryptophane B vitamin, but it won't do a bit of good if you keep thinking about those things that cause you stress. Chain smoking under stressful conditions cuts down nearly all of the vitamin C your body's moisture system needs for good health. Proper skin care requires that the mind *and* body work together to pay off.

More on Those Natural Products

The United States government allows manufacturers to claim that certain vitamins and herbals are in their products. Today's cosmetics products include fruits, vegetables, roots, herbs, and anything else commonly thought to be nutritious. The idea is that if it's good for the body it surely must be good for the skin of the face and neck. Some companies have gone almost overboard suggesting that their products are *natural*, taking cue possibly from the differences in the sales pitch made for the natural versus the synthetic vitamins. The natural, it was implied and said, is always better than the synthetic. With the natural, it was suggested, you get the real thing. There was also an implied message that the "natural" product does not cause allergic skin reactions, but that synthetic products can. Cosmetics companies will do anything to avoid saying a product is hypoallergenic—a word that angers the FDA when it's used in reference to a cosmetic product. Every cosmetic product has at least one substance that can cause an allergic reaction in somebody.

Probably in the hopes of cashing in on the back-to-nature fad in the country, some cosmetics now sally forth with flying banners claiming they are all natural, or organic. Products made from plants, foods, sea water, animal materials, and bee droppings are all over the market now, although numerous things from nature have always been used to make cosmetics. That is not really new. And natural-food products—salad oil, butter, and petrolatum—could all in many instances perform the same miracles the most expensive cosmetic moisturizers do. "But whether they are as much fun to use is up to the individual," says cosmetics lexicographer Ruth Winter, who adds: "Fancy bottles and chemicals with awesome-sounding names do not a better cosmetic make. Neither does a completely natural product necessarily offer a better result than an all-synthetic one."

Do Some Cosmetics Cost Too Much?

There are people who will pay anything if they want something badly enough. And there are those people who feel that the more something costs the better the quality will be.

The same goes for some cosmetics. Not only does one soap-making factory in the East make, package, and label soaps for many well-advertised companies, but there are cosmetics factories that save individual cosmetics firms millions of dollars by making, bottling, packaging, and labeling their skin creams and lotions for those big-name cosmetics firms, who then market and sell those products under their own names. It is not unusual for a factory to make the same product for one mass-market company to sell at $2.99 for ten ounces that it makes for another exclusive-market company to sell at fifty dollars for two ounces. The same product probably cost both companies only about twenty cents for the ingredients and about fifty cents for the package. The profit margin is enormous. The biggest expense is the magazine, newspaper, billboard, and television advertising. The exclusive store may display an elegant, appealing package, while the discount center or drugstore may display a simple bottle. But, as I have already said, it's what the particular cosmetic does for you that really counts.

One day, I picked up a plastic jar that contained eight ounces of cold cream. It cost me fifty cents at a discount store. It had an appealing label on its jar and cap. It was called Hollywood Extra Theatrical (Cleansing) Cold Cream. The label had sales phrases such as "No Makeup Kit Without It" and "Ask Any Girl on the Lot," all of which suggested that it was used by film extras. Other phrases said, "High Quality—Sensibly Priced," and "For Professional and Home Use." At other stores, the same item would or could have cost up to $1.50. And at some of the more exclusive stores, it could have cost up to twelve dollars, for it contained the same ingredients as most cold creams: mineral oil, water, parrafin, beeswax, petrolatum, ceresin, sodium borate, fragrance, methylparaben, and propylparaben. It was a product of the Devlin Pharmaceutical Company of El Segundo, California. A cheap cream? In price, yes. In quality, no. Let's face it. Cold creams are cold creams. Basically, all cold creams are cleansing creams, designed to dissolve sebum and to loosen and remove particles of dirt and other impurities. When placed on the skin, the water-soluble contents evaporate to produce a cooling effect, or "cold" feeling. Safe for any skin as long as the person using it is not allergic to one of the ingredients. Ideal for dry skin since it leaves behind a slightly oily film when it's wiped off, however, the American Medical Association and most dermatologists say that soap and water will cleanse the face just as well, and it will never cause an allergic reaction if the soap has a low pH factor.

Cold creams preceded all the current creams of the cosmetics market. The first cold cream is said to have been produced by Galen, the Greek physician, from an original formula consisting of a mixture of beeswax, water, olive oil, and rose petals. Today, the olive oil has been replaced by mineral oil, or other oils that do not easily become rancid and impure. It creates many of the same reactions on the skin as some of the best moisturizing cleansers do: it cools, removes grime and dead skin, traps in moisture, and, all in all, causes the skin to soften.

SOME SKIN-CARE PRODUCTS AND THEIR CLAIMS

Charles of the Ritz now markets its Revenescence Moist Environment Treatment line "for skin that looks like it's drenched in health." The company claims that the very active, fragrance-free, moisturizing body lotion, with added sun-screen ingredients, helps reduce chances of premature aging of the skin and skin cancer caused by overexposure to the sun. Charles of the Ritz says its Revenescence Moist Environment Body Treatment lotion contains certain moisturizers that "penetrate thirty-five cell layers!" Marketed with it is the Revenescence Moist Environment Eye Cream, "which helps soften skin and minimize lines caused by dryness."

The Charles Revson Company does very well with its C.H.R. (Charles H. Revson's initials) skin-care line. Its Ultima II series is sparked by a moisture concentrate, "A most unusual moisturizer with exclusive Collagen 100+ which helps give a more youthful look, a more supple texture to skin that is losing its elasticity." The moisture concentrate, which is applied to the skin with a circular fingertip massage action, and which prepares the skin for smooth makeup application, has an alternate, Etherea, for women allergic to the preservative parabens in the former item. C.H.R., under its Ultima II banner, has the Translucent Wrinkle Creme, a widely praised night cream. The company avows that the cream is a proven "tissue healer." It is applied at night after the skin is cleansed and toned, and is smoothed on with gentle upward and outward strokes of the fingers.

Second Debut, a product of the Beecham Company of Clifton, New Jersey, caught on as a skin-care item almost as soon as it made its counter debut. It hit the cosmetics market with good endorsements from identifiable movie actresses. The company trademarked both spellings of the name—Second Debut and 2nd Debut— and the products soared forth with a catchy tag from actress Rhonda Fleming: "Your 2nd Debut can be even better than your first." The company also offered Second Debut cleansers that "reach deep and whisk away every trace of dirt and makeup," which come in two water-soluble forms, golden liquid and whipped cream, both fortified with moisturizers and oils to leave the skin soft and dewy. This should be followed up with a skin freshener to remove traces of cleanser. Next is the 2nd Debut Facial Care Lotion, formulated with CEF (Cellular Expansion Factor) 1200. It is a pleasing and satisfying lotion, which is quickly absorbed, and which goes to work immediately to add moisture to dry skin and to plump out fine facial lines. Many women claim it is a grand daytime lotion. Then there is the Second Debut Nite-Lift, a super-rich moisturizing cream for women who prefer creams to lotions for application at night time, and who require richer moisturizing and stronger nutrients for their fragile, very dry, more mature complexions. The prices on all the Second Debut items are within most women's budgets.

Orlane, owned by the famed art collector and tomato sauce manufacturer Norton Simon, is another major cosmetics company that sells a multi-product skin-care program. It was introduced as the B-21 line, carrying a supplemental B-23 Creme to fight "against all signs of aging—fine lines, slackening of the contours, and loss of radiance." The ingredients included in Orlane's total-treatment system are powerful amino acids, vitamin A, and ingredients that attract and hold in moisture. The system can be applied over the entire body. B-23, a night cream, balances hydration, restores skin elasticity, and stimulate renewal of sluggish skin cells. It is non-occlusive, in other words, it does not stop-up skin pores.

Orlane also introduced a soon-popular Creme à la Gelée Royale Fluride, which is an organic substance featuring royal jelly, and which purportedly "helps silken wrinkles due to dryness and curb their appearance."

Miriam Bialac has a line of skin-care items that includes the Bialac Yatrolin Soap, a Haldine Firming Pick-Up, and a PABA Treatment Masque. The Bialac Yatrolin Soap contains Yatrolin Night Cream, the company claims makes the soap an effective cleanser, moisturizer, and softener. The Haldine Firming Liquid acts as "a facial muscle exerciser in the same way isometric exercises work on the body." The PABA Treatment Masque "dries and tightens the skin."

Vidal Sassoon's skin-care program is intended for morning and evening use on dry, normal, and oily skin.

The program includes an assortment of cleansing soaps and emulsions, lotion toners, and moisturizers. There is also an irrigating vitalizing lotion that flushes sluggish surface cells and stimulates new cell growth, and a Thoroughly Attentive Treatment day and night cream that lubricates excessively dry skin. Both Sassoon skincare products encourage natural color in the skin.

The Pola cosmetics are sold in numerous stores in the United States and the Orient. The firm's Eye Moisture cream is a well-known product. Called an exclusive eye-contour emollient, with a lanolin base, the Pola Eye Moisture is a mixture of Beta-Itaaman, yolk lecithin, and placenta extract. It is professed to be an outstanding penetrator. The Pola Duo Cream is called the world's first "live" multiple-vitamin cream, and is actually two creams, one aciduous and one alkaline, and both contain vitamins A, B-6, C, D-2, E, and F. Mixing the two creams simultaneously in the palm of the hand "activates" the contents to "smoothe out a roughened skin."

The "natural choice of actresses" is what some persons call the Marilyn Derigo-created Panache skin potions that sell under the name of Premiera I. The company claims the potions are used by Betty Ford, Stephanie Powers, and Alexis Smith. The Premiera line is practically all-natural and FDA-approved as "noncarcinogenic." Almond oil, and lemon, orange, and apricot oils, all cold-pressed, are included in the formulas. The company also suggests in its skin-treatment literature that "proper nutrition and exercise are an internal support to an external-care program." Bravo! Panache also offers a "Two-Week Facial Diet," a cosmetics regimen that they claim will "nourish, moisturize, and soften the skin." Most of the Panache Premiera products contain aloe vera, from the African lilylike aloe plant whose untreated juice is known for its skin-softening qualities.

In addition to the single-action line is the new, plumping Young Again wrinkle lotion, recommended on television by actress Joan Bennett. Miss Bennett declares convincingly that the lotion smoothes out facial lines and wrinkles "in three minutes," for a period of "up to eight hours." It is a mass-market item, and undoubtedly for those women who have insisted that cosmetics manufacturers produce single items designed to treat wrinkles, however temporarily. Many women do not want to follow a systematic program. They say they do not have the time or wherewithal to do this before doing that, and after following a program for ten days, they do not want to have to replenish the items.

Jheri Redding's Jhirmack Cosmetic Line, available in many beauty shops, has a wrinkle cream for the single-action crowd, although Redding insists that the entire Jhirmack line should be used "for maximum beauty and optimum results." Beauty salon attendants will assure any customer how all Jhirmack products are, in the company's opinion, superior to all other beauty and skin products, and that most Jhirmack products have a pH of 4.5 to 5.5. Redding projects his Jhirmack Wrinkle Fighter thusly: "After the age of twenty-one, most women find that the skin on the face, throat, arms, and hands begins to age more rapidly than the skin elsewhere on the body. Jhirmack has developed *pHrecedent*, a cream wrinkle fighter, which is second to none in the skin conditioning field. Blended with natural ingredients, *pHrecedent* is delicately balanced at the proper pH to help dry or aging skin. It has been designed to assist in preserving the precious qualities of a beautiful complexion." The Wrinkle Fighter, which is also sold in barber shops, sells at thirty dollars for a one-ounce jar. Its listed ingredients are water, stearic acid, glyceryl sterate, aloe, sorbitol, polysorbate 20, collagen, corn oil, mineral oil, lanolin, alcohol, procaine, hydrochloride, cetyl alcohol, benzoic acid, and vitamins E, A, and D.

Lancôme's Progrès Creme, with squalene from shark-liver oil, is one of the best moisture-holding creams. It holds in moisture while the skin is given a chance to "breathe."

One of the first temporary wrinkle lotions was Line Tamer, from Line Tamer, Inc., in Miami, although it quickly got a reputation for leaving a whitish residue. It contains water, sodium magnesium, aluminum silicate, propylene glycol, cellulose gum, and dye Red #19 and 1122.

Germaine Monteil's Supplegen Firming Action Moisture cream, Orlane's B-23 Points Vulnerable, Ultima's Creme Extraordinaire and Irma Shorell's Firming Night Creme are very effective skin-help products. But be prepared for a dent in your pocketbook. Economical is Maybelline's fairly new Moisture Whip skin-care collection.

In 1980 Elizabeth Arden began promoting its grand Millenium Face Treatment products (Hydrating Cleanser, Revitalizing Tonic, Day Renewal Emulsion and Night Renewal Creme, with paraffin masque) through facials administered in Arden's salons. The company says its Millenium Method "accelerates the natural rate of cell renewal that makes skin look, feel and function younger."

CHAPTER V

CAN SOAPS WASH AWAY SKIN PROBLEMS?

All skin is dry or oily. The only one who declares you "normal" is the psychiatrist.

Antoine Marengo

Washing cleanses, and cleansing is generally used to get rid of dirt. Exposed as it always is, the skin does get dirty. And a dirty skin is a danger in itself.

This is not to say that all skin problems have their roots in a dirty skin. Surely not, for, as we have already learned, there are numerous skin conditions that are brought on by many other causes. But in order to check or treat any skin condition or problem, and in order to get the best benefits from skin-care products, one must first cleanse the skin. It is virtually guaranteed that at whatever time of day you cleanse your skin you will find accumulated grime, grit, and common old dirt from the air, from smudgy fingertips placed on the face and from other particles and bacteria that you picked up during the day and night. And nobody will dispute that faces and necks must be cleansed before and after applications of makeup.

The big question facing women with skin problems is whether they should use soaps or chemical cleansers on their faces. Even though soap is not a cosmetic, many

105

women think of it as such, and it is considered one of the most dependable skin cleansers. Some people will use soap to cleanse the face, and will resort to chemical cleansers only when they have to remove the most stubborn and greasy makeup. On the other hand, there are women who believe soap is harmful to facial skin, and that it contains lye and other ingredients with harsh qualities inclined to sting and burn.

Oils in the skin also cause cleansing problems. In fact, natural skin oil quite often vies with dirt to make regular skin-washing a dire necessity. Oil is constantly exuded through the skin of millions of women, presenting a steady outbreak of blackheads, acne, and eczema if the skin is not kept clean. When you look at facial skin under a strong magnifying glass, you can see the immensity of these dangers as you scan the scads of little holes with oil in them. Through some of these little holes, or pores, substances may be absorbed or discharged. Fuzzy facial hair grows through some of these holes. Grit also collects in these pores, along with the oil. Until governmental hand-slapping took place, only recently, cosmetics makers advertised that their preparations could "remove excess oil from the pores of the skin and close them." No cosmetic preparation on the market can close these natural passageways without jamming in the exuding waste matter and perspiration. Such "closing" would also stop up the natural body oils nature has for nourishing and lubricating the skin surface.

For persons with dry skin, cleansing is vital because dry-skin pores are usually enlarged, and thus inviting traps for particles of dirt and cigarette smoke. These microscopic particles can cause irritation and infection if they build up in the skin.

Minute traces of skin preparations embedded in the pores can build up if they are not adequately removed.

Bacteria from perspiration, along with ever-decomposing surface cells, also build up if the skin is not moisturized regularly. The more these unwanted sediments build up in the enlarged dry-skin pores, the more inflamed the dried skin becomes. The effect can be so injurious as to require a full course of skin treatment. This is because the sedimentary buildup causes a further enlargement of the pores, causing the stem, or neck, of each pore to become narrow and impeded. This blockage can lead to many skin problems, and can make the skin thicken.

It is best to practice the "CTM" factor in caring for your skin: cleansing, toning, and moisturizing. Although many chemical skin cleansers are also astringents and toners, a separate toner is often necessary, for it perks up the skin, gives it heightened "tone," makes it feel increasingly refreshed, and removes any residue that cleansing may have left behind. Cleansing and toning alone can leave a skin high and dry. Therefore, after these two necessary procedures, moisturizing is definitely in order, to make the skin more pliant, softer, and moister. But speaking of cleansers, whatever agent you choose, it should do the following:

1. remove all dirt, grit, grime, and other residue from the skin surface
2. work non-irritatingly on your skin
3. rinse off easily and completely.

Skin cleansers come in several forms. There are soaps, cold creams, greases, lotions, and cream products that do varying kinds of cleaning jobs, some satisfactory and some less than satisfactory. There are hundreds of brands of facial soaps, from many countries, and there are more than 600 chemical cleansers.

107

Let's start with the most common and most important skin cleanser, soap.

Soap has been with us for many centuries, the initial crude types credited with making their appearance around A.D. 200. Early inhabitants of a region of Spain made castile soap, a hard, bland, generally white soap made from olive oil and glycerine.

The basic formula for soap today is an oil plus an alkali. Olive, palm, coconut, linseed, peanut, lanolin, soybean, or cottonseed oil is usually used. The alkalis, sodium hydroxide or potassium hydroxide, do most of the cleansing, but they can be quite irritating, especially to sensitive, dry skin.

Soaps cleanse the skin by first surrounding the foreign particles, and dislodging them. Water rinses them away. The rinsing must be thorough. Cake or bar soaps vary in the amount of oils or fats used. A strong soap, contains more sodium hydroxide; a mild soap is made up of chiefly fatty acids, ideal for sensitive skin, and its extra oils override any harsh alkali the soap may contain. A pleasant, almost neutral soap is one made with cold cream. Its creamy (borax and fats) base helps prevent the soap from drying out the skin. Then there is the widely used deodorant soap whose ingredients kill off bacteria that usually collect and cause perspiration odor. It is considered a bit too harsh for the face although millions suds it on their faces while showering.

There are so-called "neutral soaps," which usually have an alkaline base and a pH factor of about 10, which is somewhat high for normal skin with a pH factor of 5 to 6.5. In order to cleanse well, a soap has to have good cleansing ingredients, in other words, sodium hydroxide, which means irritation. Generally, the most popular soaps are those that are laden with oils and fatty acids, purported to relieve skin dryness because the residue left on the skin acts as an emollient.

Some of the costlier soaps combine many desirable qualities: cleansing power and lack of irritation. Paco Rabanne markets its Calandre soap, a 3.5 oz. cake, priced under five dollars, which contains the lowest possible pH and the least alkalinity. It cleanses, emulsifies, and disperses surface grime easily and rinses away thoroughly, without leaving a residue. Erno Laszlo's Special Skin Soap supposedly has similar qualities, at the same price. Etherea sells a special Oil-Control Cleansing Soap that's fragrance-free and works well on oily skin. And there's always Johnson's Baby Soap. Hard-milled and long-lasting, and devoid of strong perfumes and other allergy-arousing additives, it rinses off easily and quickly, and is ideal for adults and babies. It costs less, too. And there's always reliable, "gentle Ivory."

There are hard-water soaps, water-soluble soaps, water-activated soaps, germicidal soaps, vegetable soaps, fruit soaps, grit soaps, lemon soaps, cream soaps, and a tube-packaged cleansing cream that rinses off with water. Caswell-Massey markets a natural seaweed soap that is reputed to fight body cellulite while cleansing delicate pores. It is a natural marine soap that contains no additives or perfumes.

Whether a person wears stage or street makeup, getting the stuff off has always been a problem. Much of the makeup sold these days contains greasy substances that resist soap and that require other greasy substances, much wiping, daubing, and repeated rinsings to get them off. Good exercise for the face, but they often leave a non-emollient residue. Biotherm sells a cleansing milk, which is actually an emulsion, that easily removes makeup from water-sensitive skin, but it is not a soap.

Before leaving soaps, there are the transparent bar soaps. There are many of them, but the most popular is

Neutrogena. It is a mild soap that contains triethanolamine instead of sodium hydroxide, and it is nonalkaline. Neutrogena is also rich in glycerine. In the 1940s, as a Natone product, it was one of the first soaps in step with the fastest-growing area of cosmetics: skincare. Neutrogena provides cleansing and therapy.

In 1953, Emmanuel Stolaroff, founder of Natone Products, was in Amsterdam, Holland, when a Belgian doctor introduced him to a new soap purportedly "just right for the skin." It was a clear soap, which impressed Stolaroff. It also had high "glide" qualities because of its high glycerine content. It rinsed off easily and left no residue. And it had a pleasant fragrance. Stolaroff brought the product back to the United States, began making it, and introduced it with free samples.

"Neutrogena was the first soap to sell in American stores for a dollar," Stolaroff recounted later. "There were other glycerine soaps on the market, like Pear's Soap, but Neutrogena's formula was different. It had a nice feel and a nice smell. And it had good consumer acceptance."

Dermatologists, pediatricians, allergists, and plastic surgeons first got acquainted with Neutrogena in their offices, in their clinics, at medical meetings, and in medical journals. The medics introduced it to their patients. Today, big-selling Neutrogena is considered one of the finest skin-care soaps on the market, and a 3.5-ounce bar sells for only slightly above the debut price of one dollar.

Soaps can be good cleansing agents if they are the *right* soaps. The "wrong" soaps do not do what you want them to satisfactorily and non-irritatingly. Some "wrong" soaps present problems for some types of facial skin by awakening all kinds of allergic conditions, and even make dry skin drier and more irritated. Some will drive a woman with oily skin to alcohol cleansers, which may cause more troubles.

We should never forget, however, that soap is primarily a cleaning agent. It can never be an effective skin-*treatment* product, regardless of what is put in it, and even the mildest soap for the face can be used too much. Some people with oily skin wash their faces three or four times a day, afraid that oily skin is akin to disaster. Loofahs and Buf-Pufs can be used instead of soap at times to rub off flaky, shedding skin, and for dry skin this is probably best, for soap in its mildest state can often irritate ultra-dry skin. Some women with oily skin who wash several times daily with soap complain that no matter how many times a day they dive into those ablutions, their skin is still oily, sometimes more so. It's possible that the frequent washing actually increases the sebum action. In such cases, reduce the frequency of the washing, and use a good astringent after you wash. If you are going to be putting on makeup, use Clinique's Pore-Minimizer Makeup. Do not get the idea that this will permanently shrink your pores; nothing will do that. But temperature, hot and cold water, and various astringents will make your pores enlarge and tighten, temporarily.

Like cold cream, one of the world's oldest non-soap facial cleansers, almost all the scores of chemical face cleaners on the market contain mineral oil. Borax gives most of them their cleaning power, with detergents packed in to make it easier for rinsing to whisk off any residue. Most of the more familiar facial cleansers, whether they are creams, lotions, or greases, have oil-base formulas that perform like solvents on makeup and surface skin oils. Some of the cleansers have emulsifying ingredients that break down dirt, oil, and grease so that they wash off easily with lukewarm water. Most women who wear cosmetics have for years used wipe-

111

off cleansers, followed by soap and water washings, tonings, and recently moisturizers. The wipe-off cleansers used to be of the cold cream or Albolene cream variety—grease to knock off grease. But in recent years, cleansers have become more dainty, less messy, and thankfully more efficient. And they rinse off. But even these new facial cleansers contain many of the same ingredients that were in the old-time cleansers. This has made cosmetics makers inject "extra" and pleasant-sounding ingredients into their newer, daintier cleansers, like "fat-free milk" and "whipped" and "medicated" substances.

To begin with, no woman today likes to use a "grease" cleaner on her face. Women don't like having greasy hands, wiping cloths, and skin. Nor do they like the greasy feeling they are left with. This is quite often the complaint of women who have used cold creams and other greaselike products, called liquefying creams, which become like liquefied oil when they are rubbed on the skin. They sit on the skin for a few minutes, causing it to perspire, and then the cream, the makeup, and the dirt are all wiped off. Even a thorough wiping with a dry cloth, cotton, gauze, or towel will seldom wipe off all the liquefied oil, as some of it sinks into the skin's pores and settles there until sebum, more perspiration, or a strong chemical cleanser flushes it out, usually after first dissolving it.

Over the years, that kind of messiness has paved the way for the acceptance of myriad non-liquefying cleansing creams and lotions. The more convenient a cleanser is to apply and remove, the more women prefer it. Of course, some women prefer a cleanser that they feel is best for their individual skin type, or a product that is more effective than others in removing makeup. Mascara can be stubborn when confronted by some cleansers, yet fades quickly with others. Some

112

women do not like gooey cleansers, and others dislike runny ones. Some customers prefer a cleanser that not only removes dirt and makeup, but that also removes flaky skin. They would rather not use a separate facial scrub scream. Cleansers cannot be everything, although some of them try to be. And cleansers, like soap, are not treatment items, unless they are germicidal soaps and cleansers. Cleansers are only for cleansing.

There are fragrance-free cleansers for those who dislike scents, for not everybody loves the smell of cold cream. Harsh cleansers often cause a reaction in super-sensitive skin, calling for "gentle agents" such as milk-base lotions and "organic" cleansing milks. There is something for everybody.

We could examine numerous brands and kinds of facial cleansers, and I probably could go on forever outlining their unique qualities. But as I have already noted, there are more than 600 facial cleansers on the market.

The important thing to bear in mind in selecting any facial cleanser, and using it, is how thoroughly it cleanses your skin. Always use common sense. If the cleanser is the kind that rinses off, be sure to rinse it off. You'd be surprised how many unthinking women will use a rinsable cleanser on their faces and wipe it off with facial tissues instead of rinsing it off. This often causes traces of the cleanser to be left on the skin, covering dirt left in the pores and subsequently creating an irritative buildup. Excess sebum results, and the skin becomes sore. And this can cause pores to enlarge from infection.

CHAPTER VI

TREATS, TREATMENTS and THERAPEUTICS

No one is perfect and no one ever will be. Minor imperfections never stop those who are determined to improve on their lot.

Jack LaLanne, *Abundant Health & Vitality After 40*

According to *Town & Country* magazine, Beverly Hills is a golden ghetto of 34,000 residents where, among other things, psychiatrists and plastic surgeons abound and beauty buffs spend four hundred dollars each week to be "made up" twice daily, and "where at twenty-five you're over the hill, and looking young is the only form of Social Security that really counts." Beverly Hills is only one geographical area, but at least its beauty-conscious ladies believe in something—cosmetics, skin care, and themselves.

There is nothing wrong in believing in the power of a chemical solution to transform a tired face into one full of glowing vitality and beauty. If the advertising says this or that commodity will do it, the buyer has half the battle won just by believing what the advertising says. The other half of the battle depends on how the product is used. Often, the trusting buyer/user is beautifully rewarded with results that are both visibly and mentally positive. Occasionally, some users find that certain products do not do what the advertisers claim. Needless to say, those users who find some products effective become lifetime customers of the products, and those meeting with ineffectiveness drop the item and seek something else. They will ask cosmetics specialists, keep ears open for positive comments from friends, read magazine and newspaper ads, and try, try again. It's sad but some of these women never find the "right" thing. Maybe they want a new face overnight. Maybe they are looking for something for somebody else's face, and don't know it. Maybe it's too late for a "temporary" cream or lotion or full-course treatment to make any significant changes in a skin assaulted by years of sun, inattention, hereditary factors, and a depressed state of mind.

Women who believe in themselves do not wait until they are fifty to begin taking care of their skin. Women who believe in themselves set a regimen and live by it; they pay attention to all the things that have to do with their beauty, diets, and minds. No woman given to whimsy and constant indecision can stick to any one thing long enough to even notice results, positive or negative. It takes a strong and methodical mind to conclude what the condition is, what is needed to help it, and to seek the right thing to help it. For this woman, an expensive full-course beauty treatment is often a treat worth waiting for.

Surely, no woman wants to buy six jars of an expensive skin treatment if she can buy one product, at any cost, that will do the same job. But hardly anything on the market will do that. The most popular fine-line elixirs demand that supplemental products be used, too. Lately, it appears that good skin care also demands a change in one's diet, physical exercise for the face and body, and an improved mental state. Vitamins geared to the specific skin conditions are also recommended. No one cosmetic is the fountain of youth, or is it going to remove facial lines and wrinkles permanently. But lines and wrinkles can be retarded, or avoided. Wrinkles can be suppressed, erased, and banished without plastic surgery. Just as some medical people disdain chiropractors, so, too, some plastic surgeons discount any skin remedies except their own. Some dermatologists recoil at the thought of a cosmetic doing what they believe only drugs should do. But the public demands results. Who delivers is of no consequence. Personally, I have found that certain cosmetics work wonders as they tone, de-oil, firm, smooth, and invigorate my skin. Some give temporary, some lasting, results. For thin lines and painful hickies around my chin, a 100 mg of RNA/DNA taken daily removes them in less then three weeks, makes my face livelier, and energizes my body. PABA, folic acid, and B-Coms-50 put color into my skin and hair, and, combined with castor-oil massages, remove mild discolorations. A selective diet and a pleasant mental disposition help. As I mentioned earlier, I do not recommend prolonged use of any "wrinkle-removing" lotion or cream. In time, the stuff only accents wrinkles and lines.

All of us, however, are different in more ways than anyone could ever imagine. To one woman, an austere regimen is the answer, one calling for a meager use of cosmetics, a fasting diet, restrained exercise, and no vitamins. To another woman, an abundance of cosmetics fill the bill, too many to keep on a dresser top, in a medicine chest, on the back of a water closet, or in a closet case; scads of all kinds of vitamins; liberal quantities of "rest" pills; no exercise that's not up to the par of Jack LaLanne's; and a strict vegetarian diet. A load of contradictions and countereffects. Often the "progress" is measurable only by the individual woman.

Some women believe they can rid their eyes of puffiness by sleeping with their heads sharply elevated. Some women desperately try to remove broken capillaries beneath their skin by "baptizing" the areas several times a day with alcoholic astringents. Heaven forbid. Some women believe that sleeping under a coating of Vaseline or cold cream will make their skin sweat, thus removing a need for moisturizers. They never manage to cleanse the goo fully from their pores, and if they do, they have scrubbed their faces raw in the process, necessitating use of several other emollients to soothe and correct the secondary condition.

Some women believe that as they grow older their skin muscles find it more and more difficult to withstand the forces of gravity, not knowing that as we grow older our entire bodies get in this fight. That is why there is nothing we can do to our faces alone that will suffice in this quest for skin beauty. The victors find the battle is won from within and without.

Considering that some advertisers claim that this or that cosmetic can "penetrate the layers of the skin," it is no wonder that so many women believe that their cosmetics do just that and remedy conditions from deep down. But dermatologists swear that the skin's dead layer on top of the epidermis is about as far as any cosmetic penetrant will go. In fact, they declare, if cosmetics contained chemicals that could go through the skin layers and thus change body conditions, they would not be cosmetics but drugs. Counter cosmetics do not have the abilities of ultraviolet rays. When an astringent "plumps" the skin, it makes the skin pucker, makes the pores rush together, close ranks, and get smaller to ward off anything coming next. As soon as the effects of the astringent wear off, usually in a few hours, the pores return to normal and the puckered smoothness is gone.

Dr. Barbara Gilchrest, a staff dermatologist at Boston's Beth Israel Hospital and a Harvard Medical School instructor, says we can expect only short-term benefits from most skin-care products on the market today. "Moisturizers," says Dr. Gilchrest, "can make your skin feel more comfortable; cosmetics can make you look better. But you experience the benefits only on the day you use the product . . . You could use a moisturizer every day of your life and your skin wouldn't be any different than if you hadn't used it."

If what Dr. Gilchrest says is true, women should not seek a one-bottle cure-all for lines or wrinkles, but should look for a product that can provide a temporary change. After all, cosmetics are in themselves superficial, or "on the surface." They make you *look* good, and when you look good, you *feel* good. For any lasting or real change, I suggest an overall approach, as outlined throughout this book.

As you try to ward off the appearance of aging, surely you should bear in mind that the condition did not come about solely from outside factors, or just to the face. Many factors play a role in creating facial conditions, and they do not do it overnight. Aging is a progressive state, brought on by heredity, worry, bad diet, a lack of body and facial exercises, a deficiency in the number of fertilizing enzymes in the immune system, and all too often a negative attitude. The sun does its part, too.

Something I think worth studying is the increasing belief that mental attitudes can actually influence body molecules for better or worse. The mind has amazing powers, many still not understood.

The gods alone do not age, wrote Sophocles, more than 2,000 years ago. Mortal men and mortal women do not have such a luxury. We humans two-step through life with a seemingly measured cadence, our every phase orchestrated by a conductor apparently unsympathetic to our dislike of a mellow cantabile called aging. Probably people would not mind aging if the process did not connote deterioration. Because it does, many men and women will not listen when someone compliments them by saying a wrinkle or a line here and there gives a look of wisdom and maturity to the face. If they are told facial massaging and toning will help ward off and remedy lines and wrinkles, they are immediately thrown into confusion by statements of plastic surgeons that massaging and toning are not good for the skin and that they will do no good. Damned if they do and damned if they don't.

How appealing to some women the following ad looks in a magazine:

AT WHAT AGE DO YOU START TO LOOK LIKE AN "OLDER WOMAN"?

Pretty scary, isn't it? How quickly you can go from looking young to looking like an "older woman." It's almost as if one day you wake up and there they are—those tiny lines and wrinkles that tell the world your age. Or worse, make you look older than you are. Yes, it's a shock. But it's a shock that we all face sooner or later. And yes, there is something we can do to help. There is a unique beauty fluid that women all over the world have discovered. Here in the United States, it is called Oil of Olay. . . . Make Oil of Olay part of your beauty regimen, starting today. Once you've discovered the secret of Oil of Olay, you've discovered the secret of younger-looking skin.

119

The foregoing is from an Oil of Olay one-page advertisement that appeared in the highly circulated *Family Circle* magazine. Its headline is immediately catching, and its text is instantly understandable and appealing to any reader concerned about "age signs." Overall, the ad tells how Oil of Olay is "greaseless," how it "penetrates so quickly," and how it works with natural body fluids "to restore your own youthful moisture balance." Other catchy phrases tell how Oil of Olay eases dryness that causes lines and wrinkles, softens and smooths skin, and brings out a natural glow.

How can any concerned woman resist such declarations? Few can resist, for Oil of Olay is one of the biggest skin-softening products on the cosmetics market. Four ounces sell for about three dollars. Like Doak's Formula 405, Revlon's Milk Plus Six, Raintree by Noxzema, Gillette's Deep Magic, Norcliff-Thayer's Esoterica, and the creams by Keri and Nivea, Oil of Olay sells on the mass market massively. It is apparent that there is a great need for these products, most of which do make the skin more youthful-looking and softer, however only temporarily. Most women who use the products say they do what they say they will, if one keeps using them. Who can find fault with that except someone seeking to be born again?

Cosmetics makers have been in the forefront for years, offering products designed to camouflage or soften and diminish signs of aging. If only our scientists were able to make us live longer and grow older gracefully without the signs of aging being imprinted on our faces!

Gerontologists, scholars who study the aging process, say we are tending to live longer, because of vast improvements in medical care, and scientists are testing Gerovital, the Roumanian drug derived from Novocain, the dental anesthetic, and said by many advocates to do a lot to rejuvenate aging persons. At the University of California, research into the cellular mechanisms involved in aging now indicate that if aging cannot be totally suppressed then at least its onset might be delayed and its harsher signs softened.

Is wrinkle-causing aging the result of the breakdown of body cells, or a proscribed genetic process programmed differently for each individual according to her and his heredity? Another question under study is how our diet affects the signs of aging.

Medical laboratories are working overtime to determine the roles of enzymes, hormones, the endocrine glands, and cellular molecules, studying interrelated processes that, like chain reactions, lead to organic breakdowns. Medical research has disclosed that although some parts of our bodies reproduce cells throughout our lives, in order to heal a bruise or cut, for example, there is a cessation of cell reproduction at certain times in our muscles, brain, and heart. Melanocytes, which manufacture melanin for protection against sunburn, cease manufacturing melanin at certain stages in our lives. This is extremely bad for very fair-skinned persons who, already had a decreased supply of melanin-producing melanocytes at birth.

As body cells deteriorate, new cells generally form, but in order for a cell to multiply, it must divide, and each part find its own place and function prescribed by heredity. As we age, cells lose their ability to multiply and also their ability to decode specific instructions during synthesis of protein. The firming qualities of collagen are lost. The natural protein of the skin, which gives the skin its youthful suppleness and elasticity, is no longer being synthesized. As a result, the facial skin begins to sag and droop. Since gerontological science has not yet come up with a suitable remedy, it has be-

121

come the task of dermatologists working with major cosmetics makers to devise and concoct cosmetic solutions, however transitory the benefits may be.

Dr. Paul Niehans, the eminent pioneer in the study of live-cell therapy, struggled for many years in Montreux, Switzerland, trying to retard the inevitable process of aging. He conceived a revolutionary medical technique of injecting fresh, living cells from a special breed of fetal black-mountain sheep to regenerate aging human organs. Dr. Niehans had found that the cells of the sheep were rich in vitamin B-1, which made the sheep highly resistant to cancer. Patients injected with this live-cell formula said they had new-found vigor and a feeling of fitness they remembered only from their younger years. According to reports, their faces also showed a new radiance and firmness. From these experiments rose the now-famous La Prairie Clinic, located on the edge of Lake Geneva in the Alpine foothills, which has admitted and treated more than 60,000 patients since it began.

From the famed La Prairie Clinic came the now popular La Prairie skin-care preparations—selected substances based on Dr. Niehan's live-cell treatment. The preparations, in cream bases and on sale in finer stores around the world, made their official United States debut in 1979, when it was announced that "La Prairie opens up exciting possibilities for preserving the skin's youthful beauty" and helps to "stave off the ravages of stress and aging." It was further stated that "all La Prairie preparations are infused with preserved embryonic cell extracts in the form of full placental tissue," and that all La Prairie selected products contain elastin and collagen. The latter ingredient was first introduced into cosmetics in stabilized and soluble form by Germaine Monteil.

Monteil, which has long enjoyed an exalted reputation in the American cosmetics marketplace, still includes elastin and collagen in its big-selling Supplegen line of beauty treatments.

In most instances, it is moisturizing that is emphasized as an aid for dry facial skin. Many cosmetics companies stress moisturizing qualities in their impressive assortment of creams and lotions. Advertising copywriters conjure up phrases to project the message that these cosmetics can retard weathered and depressed conditions on the faces of American men and women. Moisture and more moisture, the messages scream. It is amazing how long it took for Americans to wake up to the fact that their skin thrives on moisture.

After cleansing and toning, most women consider a good moisturizer essential. Moisture keeps the skin cells plump and wellshaped. When moisture is not retained, the skin cells lose whatever shape they have and show up on the epidermis as lines and wrinkles.

Men and women use many means and products to make their skin produce moisture. Aside from the petroleum jellies and cold creams, they use heat spas, dry steam baths, heated bedrooms, heat pads, heat blankets, heat corsets, heat vibrators, and heat face masks. Baseball pitcher Nolan Ryan once told a Los Angeles radio commentator that he uses a rubber "sleeve" on his pitching arm. He said the device causes his arm to develop inner heat, making it generate moisture, which causes the overworked arm to avoid muscular contraction and stiffness. Heat builds up moisture, which in turn induces softness, suppleness, and vitality.

Imperial Formula is one cosmetic line that promotes moisture retention in its wrinkle-treatment package. Imperial assures that its Bio-Protective Moisture System penetrates the skin instantly. It is light and nongreasy, and should be used under Imperial Formula's Liquid Pro-X Moisture Lotion, which provides "a dewy cushion to enable smoother application of makeup." Some wrinkle treatments create a glassy condition on the surface of the skin, making makeup application difficult. It's like trying to apply oil paint to a water-wet surface. But Imperial Formula's Wrinkle Concentrée applied in droplets to lined areas of the face makes for easy makeup application. For regular treatment of lines and wrinkles, Imperial offers its emollients: Nutricia F99, Special Eye Cream and Extra-Rich Throat Cream F53.

An emollient, in any consistency, should remain on the skin for a specific period of time, usually overnight. Most emollients are a mixture of oils. If the oils are the low-melting kind, they will usually feel greasy on the skin. Just the opposite is the case if they are of the high-melting kind. They disappear quickly, leaving a smooth feeling on the skin. But any benefits usually come not from the oils but from the water in the emollients, as water is known to soften the skin. That is why a person whose feet sweat all the time seldom complains of calluses, a somewhat hereditary condition that is more common among people whose feet stay dry all the time. Emollients minimize the loss of natural moisture from the skin. The night emollients usually have vitamin A in them to keep the skin resilient and supple. Glycerine is sometimes added because it can draw moisture from the air. Ancient emollients always contained rose water, beeswax, and glycerine—ingredients found in some emollients even today.

Really good emollients do help soften the skin and make it feel smoother. They reduce flaking, roughness, and irritation, and there is ample evidence that these mild balms actually aid in retarding fine lines and wrinkles. That's probably why there are so many emollients on the market, in all sizes and in all prices, everywhere, in everything. A woman I know was aghast one day when she walked into a discount drugstore and saw a big display of Jean Naté moisturizing lotion, nineteen ounces for three dollars. She had just bought a four-ounce moisturizer at Neiman-Marcus for twelve dollars. "And they both contain the same ingredients!" she wailed.

Some treatments are for daytime and others for nighttime. They come in many varieties for all types of skin. Lancaster of Monaco's Suractif, called "the most important advance in skin care since moisturizers," is a skin program offered in finer stores. Lancaster Cosmetics acclaim that their anti-wrinkle course "actually aids the skin's natural ability to renew itself."

Lancaster's price structure for its skin treatment line instantly took the product out of the mass market. The Active Day Treatment was introduced at forty-five dollars; Night Treatment seventy-five dollars; Throat Treatment fifty dollars; Eye Treatment forty-five dollars, and Oil Treatment thirty-five dollars.

Estée Lauder's Swiss Performing Extract is acclaimed as a penetrating, collagenated moisturizer the company and customers say rejuvenates skin cells. It made its counter debut at forty dollars for 3 3/4 ounces. Estée Lauder's European Performing Creme is used in conjunction with the Swiss Performing Extract. The latter product goes on first for women with normal skin, day or night, and for women with dry skin. Then the European Performing Creme goes over with pearly white, greaseless smoothness, functioning in several ways to provide maximum moisturizing and minimal lubrication. It supposedly protects the skin from damage caused by stress, abuse, and air pollution, and also prevents moisture loss. The company vows that this product increases the skin's capacity to retain more moisture through the use of a special, complex formula that is highly hygroscopic (readily taking up and retaining moisture), and that it also allows the skin to "breathe." It is usually used after cleansing and toning, and is applied sparingly over the face and throat until it is absorbed. The company urges that people with normal and dry skin fare better if European Performing Creme is used over a primary application of Swiss Performing Extract. Used in this way, the company declares, "tiny dehydration lines disappear or become much less visible, and under makeup it provides a moist and dewy look instead of an oily shine . . . With repeated use, your skin stays soft and smooth."

Lauder's Maximum Care Eye Creme is for use on all types of skin, and is guaranteed by the company to erase fine lines around the eyes, if used regularly. It never creases or cakes with makeup. It contains natural soluble protein to help the skin around the eyes stay young-looking, and it contains vitamin E and avocado oil.

Then there is Estée Lauder's well-known Re-Nutriv, which came out a few years back at $115, and in the inflationary days of 1980 was selling for only about fifteen dollars more. It is known as an anti-wrinkle cosmetic.

Several companies market special "wrinkle stick" treatment items for convenient carrying and quick, easy application. Some of the stick applicators appear in the skin-care lines of Ultima, Clinique, Etherea, and De Markoff, and sell at around $6.50.

Clinique, a Lauder subsidiary, has a Sub-Skin Cream that fits into a special Clinique skin routine and is recommended for use on fine, dry facial lines. How does Sub-Skin Cream work? "Amazingly," avers Clinique. "Put it on your own clean, bare skin, and you don't even have to be patient. The cream sinks in immediately, *works on and within the skin* adding a special kind of collagen extract that actually penetrates many layers of skin. Soluble collagen, it is believed, accounts for much of the skin's elasticity and firmness. . . . The collagen in this cream is unusually effective, and took many years to develop and test. Clinique Sub-Skin Cream represents a major advance in the care of fine-lined skin—*it's the most updated cream available today. It gets results.*"

Elizabeth Arden's Bye-Lines is a complete program in one container for people who "worry about wrinkles-to-come, or about skin that's loose and lined." By-Lines is a sheer, clear, light wrinkle lotion for use under makeup. It is an all-day lotion advertised to help smooth out "those little time-lines that give away honest age." The lotion lets makeup go on with ease. Arden also has a Bye-Lines Replenishing Lotion with its own trademark ingredient Elastigen 400, plus a Bye-Lines Replenishing Throat Cream and Nightcare Cream for Eyes, which also contains Elastigen 400 and a blend of tea (internodes of Oriental astringent leaves used by natural cosmeticians to reduce puffiness around eyes), myristoyl, hydrolyzed animal protein, squalane, avocado oil, and emollient esters (an ester is a compound of aciduous alcohol from which water has been extracted; the fragrant liquids are used for artificial fruit perfumes and flavors).

But Arden's biggest push is behind its Visible Difference, which the company calls an intensive moisture-penetration system. It comes in three forms: Visible Difference Special Moisture-Formula for BodyCare, Visible Difference Refining Moisture-Creme Complex (for the face), and Visible Difference Eyecare Concentrate. Large, small and smaller. The large size is for the body, and the smaller container is for the eyes. Arden stresses that a companion commodity be used on the whole body, although few people develop noticeable lines and wrinkles below their necks.

127

In promoting the qualities of its Visible Difference products, Arden outlines "the results of some of the many carefully monitored tests that were conducted by the Elizabeth Arden Laboratories to prove the unique performance and effectiveness of Visible Difference's deep moisture penetration." Photographs taken by an electron microscopic camera show how surface skin changed after Visible Difference was applied for twenty-one days. Arid, depressed skin looks voluptuous, with the skin pillowed and cushioned with moisture. *"Proof,"* says Arden, "that continued use promotes a visible, tested, measureable difference in the skin's surface." Arden stressed also that tests with the Visible Difference eye cream showed that marked results were evident "in just three hours!" Also emphasized was Arden's claim that Visible Difference "penetrates almost to where new skin [epidermis] is born. As much as twenty-five cell layers deep depending on regional thickness of the skin."

It must be noted, however, that "twenty-five cell layers" is not comparable to "twenty-five skin layers." Thousands of "cell layers" may look like a thick blanket under a microscope, but under the naked eye they could look like the thinnest tissue paper, or the depth of the outer layer of the usually dead skin lying atop the epidermis, which normally replaces itself every twenty-eight days anyway. Such claims do get attention, however, and make sales blossom. With all the emphasis on penetration, people should begin to realize that changes must happen beneath the surface of the skin to do any good. But help for the skin does not only come from within the body either. That's why it pays to find cosmetics that will do our skin the most good cosmetically, in terms of appearance and surface health. We also must follow living and dietary patterns that will help our bodies as entities and enrich our skin. For a woman who foolishly spends most of her daytime hours under the sun, her skin unprotected, there is no cosmetic product that will remove or adequately hide the resultant damage. Cosmetics, used steadily and faithfully, can ameliorate some of the surface damage after a while, and they can help moisturize the arid skin after a while, or give the appearance that they have helped. Selective vitamins can probably help bring on enzymic changes that can re-stimulate collagenic fibers and cellular regeneration in aging skin. Cosmetic moisturizers and skin texturizers can go to work on the surface of such skin, and visible changes *will* take place, helped, of course, by constant facial exercises of the kind obtained from your own at-home face lift. So much desperation can be avoided in mid-life and later life if a woman begins early in life to take good care of her skin.

With so many moisturizers on the market today, one could safely surmise that all women have dry skin and that most women have trouble getting their skin to act or look right because there is not enough natural moisture in it to prevent flakiness, scaliness, lines, and wrinkles. In some cases, that could be true, but not in all. Some women at sixty have plenty of moisture in the skin of their faces and necks, but find their elbows and shins ashen and dry. There are other women, who for years have been known as so-called "outdoor" types, whose bodies had a supple softness but whose faces long ago took on such a glazed look that the apt treatment would be turtle wax, not turtle oil. All of this proves that women must learn what kind of skin they have, what its deficiencies and good points are, whether soap and water is best or a particular cosmetic cleanser and toner, and whether to use or avoid concoctions containing alcohol, lanolin, oils, or whatever. Maybe the "irritative" qualities of a certain cosmetic are not "working on" your skin and "doing it good," but actually irritating it because you are allergic to some chemical ingredient in the cosmetic. This is where most women "shelf buyers" get into trouble. They feel automatically condemned to trial-and-error testing, and sometimes do further damage to their skin. This can be avoided if you consult a qualified, knowledgeable cosmetics specialist. The so-called finer stores, or finer cosmetics counters, have such specialists. Any reputable dermatologist acquainted with current-market cosmetics can also be counted on to help. In the chapter "Your Regimen for a Beautiful Skin," I will discuss how to ascertain which cosmetics are best for you, how they are to be used, when, and for how long.

Lancôme is another innovative cosmetics company. Sold worldwide, its products are available in 130 countries. Throughout the years, the firm has been a pioneer in the cosmetics industry. Lancôme discovered how to stablize the serum in treatment creams, a way of incorporating DNA (deoxyrlbonucleic acid, the basic substance of all cell life) into a product; how vitamins can be used in normalizing and regenerative creams, and how cellular and sea-water extracts can be used.

It was back in 1936 that Lancôme, based in France, brought out its Nutrix Balancing Night Cream and its Adieu Rides ("Goodbye Lines") Eye Creme, making it possible for women to minimize dry skin and expression lines. In 1972, Hydrix was introduced as Lancôme's "moisture trap," which trapped in skin moisture day and night. Customers swear by Lancôme's Progrés lotion, a blend of smoothing emollients, moisturizers, and humectants (substances used to preserve moisture contents), including active collagen. Progrés makes the skin "lie down," softening it without disturbing its natural functions. Progrés draws in moisture while forming a barrier against escape, or evaporation, from the skin.

Progrés is also an affirmed skin "plumper," a gentle but sure taskmaster for dried-out surface cells. Lancôme's Absolue is another item well worth noting. It is a multi-property night cream for all types of skin, and the first cream to contain DNA, which increases the cell's capacity to reproduce, and thus slows down the aging process and speeds up the chances for formation of new, young cells. Absolue makes wrinkles and light scars lie low, it is contended by the company, and hydrates and normalizes the skin when applied nightly. The eye cream Adieu Rides minimizes laugh lines at the corners of the eyes, and smooths away crepiness. Lecithin, a known skin softener, is included in its ingredients.

It has not been long since women first began to think of cosmetics in terms of "treatments." Before, most women were interested merely in makeup. A dab of this after a smudge of that after use of an alcoholic skin cleanser or following a general ablution of a petrolatum cleansing cream and away they'd go. Only a few years ago, women began to make their own skin treatments, using items selected from various sources and for certain purposes. Then along came the age of physical fitness, body-changing diets, and the makeup secrets of the movie and television stars. Columnists disclosed the skin-care practices of notable women, and other women read these disclosures and said to themselves, "There but for the grace of something, go I." News also became more widespread, especially via television, of facial and bodily changes wrought by plastic surgery. No longer was somebody's face lift, decreased hips, or displaced derriere a hush-hush topic. Betty Ford marched into every woman's home via newspaper, magazine, and television with news of her surgical face lift. At once, thousands of women began to want similar facial transformations without surgery. If Dr. Jeckyl could drink a special potion and become a horrendous Mr. Hyde, why couldn't Penelope Schultz eat or drink something that could transform her face into that of a beauty? Why not one thing, or a series of things, that could merely be applied to the face periodically to bring about beautiful changes? Since we supposedly live in an age of wonders, why shouldn't there be magical facial aids to banish lines, suppress wrinkles, and give someone a refreshing new face without making her look as if she forgot to take off the Linit mask? Cosmetics manufacturers had heard these questions for a long time. They were becoming louder and more numerous. Something had to be done quickly. To the laboratories they headed, emerging with treatments rather than singular treats. They called the public's attention to these new cosmetics discoveries through massive advertising campaigns. Avon stepped up its door-to-door sales activities, thrusting into millions of feminine hands colorful brochures depicting its Vita-Moist creams and lotions. Sales aces in top stores were called into seminars to learn the face-saving attributes of scores of new synergistic skin-care systems, programs, and plans. Inquisitive customers were told warmly and methodically what the benefits of this lotion were when used in combination with that cream, under certain conditions at a particular time of day or night, and on normal, dry, or oily skin. Promising results made the cosmetics sound, look, and feel exciting. And so many women needed promising results quickly. It had become suddenly evident that millions of women had spent most of their lives taking hit-and-miss care of their faces, giving more attention to makeup than to skin care. Not unusual, probably, when you consider that most people wait until a skin condition becomes crucial before they seek help for it. Physicians have been trying for years to get people to get medical attention often, to engage in preventive medicine, so that any untoward condition can be caught and checked before it becomes serious. But so many people feel that anything they do not see is not there and probably never will be there. But change is constant, and often invisible. Our mind's eye is not a time-lapse camera, capable of showing the steady growth of change. When we generally see a change, it is already painfully there. That's when panic sets in. Anything to erase these lines! Anything to soften this crusty skin!

Not only are women becoming more conscious of the available skin-care systems and new solutions for various skin conditions, but they are also centering their attention on skin-treatment products that have been on the market for years—cosmetic programs they thought were "playthings" used only by rich old ladies and aging movie stars.

Recently, the fifty-year-old Erno Laszlo skin-care regimen began to get attention from women who had always thought it was beyond their means. The housewife who learned it was proper to pay three hundred dollars to buy a new set of tires for her car began to realize that it was just as sensible to pay two hundred dollars for facial treatments that would possibly make her look a lot better.

The root of the Laszlo beauty technique is the pH factor—acid versus alkaline. Every Laszlo product has a "pH factor." Any chemistry student has learned that the pH signifies a degree of acidity or alkalinity. In the Laszlo regimen, pH is not the name of a chemical ingredient, nor some miraculous skin-transforming drug. It is simply an eye-catching and thought-provoking term suggesting a balance in the skin's natural acids. Laszlo suggests that it is important to maintain a certain level of acidity to acquire and keep beautiful skin. Laszlo says an "acid mantle" protects the skin from ever-dangerous pollutants and bacteria in the air. This, by the way, is the same position taken by Paula Meehan's Redken Labs in advertisements for their skin-conditioning products, sold in thousands of beauty shops. Both Laszlo and Redken maintain that this acid mantle can be shattered and penetrated by certain cosmetics containing alkaline ingredients that let in wrinkle-causing germs.

Laszlo stresses proper cleansing of the skin, urges diligent testing of cosmetic products for alkalinity, and encourages customers to shun those products containing alkaline chemicals. One thing quite memorable about Dr. Laszlo is his contention, quoted throughout the years, about washing. When an elderly woman is asked how she kept her skin wrinkle-free into her eighties, she often announces flatly that she's had a life-long habit of washing her face daily with water. Dr. Laszlo once said that the reason cosmetics companies seldom suggest this is because they've never found a way to make a profit from water.

One of the fortes of the Erno Laszlo Institute is that it sends its finely trained staff of sales consultants to finer stores to explain Laszlo's colorful skin-care rituals and the benefits of the numerous Laszlo soaps, creams, lotions, powders, and oils. Customers using the Laszlo course must buy the entire treatment package, at a cost in early 1980 of approximately $150.

Some companies have treatments, others programs, and still others skin systems. Payot of Paris offers its skin-care products in a series. Payot Facialistics are marketed as "a health club for your face." There are Payot skin-care salons all over the world, even in Venezuela. Payot products are provided not just by skin type, but by age. Payot prescribes a three-step at-home daily facial consisting of seven easy facial massage movements, four facial exercises, and specified treatment products. Payot's products are not just applied, but *massaged* into the skin. The massaging is one of the main differences between Payot's cosmetics and others, and it is emphasized strongly in its sales approach. In a way, it sort of revives a practice that was used extensively in the past, but that was abandoned during the last ten to twenty years. Men often used to get massages in barber shops. The barbers would use their fingers and electrified Oster hand massagers; apply herbal solutions, mud packs, and astringents to the customer's face, along with blistering hot towels laid over the face to moisturize the skin, soften it, and start the blood circulating. The intermittent but frequent massaging did the rest to make the man's skin feel a thousand times better than it had the previous week. In those days, women, too, would visit barbers for the same massages, but these women were often thought to be a bit mannish. Only a few of the beauty shops afforded facial massages of the same type. The late Eddie Senz, noted facial and makeup expert for years on New York's East Side, built up much of his clientele among wealthy New York women by providing facials and images for actresses Jayne Meadows, Rita Gam, Lena Horne, and stars of the Metropolitan Opera. When Helena Rubinstein was alive, she often stressed the importance of daily face massage, although few cosmetics people today stress massaging. Barber shops started disappearing some years back when men began wearing their hair long. Ritzier shops bloomed, most of them concentrating on newer, "mod" styles for men, and little attention was given to skin. Most men were interested chiefly in growing their hair, or having hair implanted. For many men, the more rugged their faces looked the better.

Many women in today's rushing world do not have the time to massage their faces twice daily. Maybe at night, after work, and before retiring, but in the morning, they are rushing to hit the freeway or subway to get to work. There is no time for massages. Probably that is

135

why the Payot line is mainly in highly exclusive and monied areas where the stores cater to women of leisure—in Beverly Hills, in Detroit's Grosse Pointe, along Miami's Gold Coast, in Pasadena's San Marino, and in the wealthier districts of other major American cities. Women in these areas have the time to massage their faces all day, and the money to hire somebody else to do it for them.

For her majesty of the evening only, Payot suggests: "Your skin can enjoy the luxury of daily massage in the evening, as you apply the night cream recommended for your skin type. Massage it into the skin, *repeating each movement three to five times*. (1) Muscles are strengthened, toned, and firmed; (2) Blood circulation is activated, giving skin a freshness and a glow; (3) Skin is softened, smoothed, and moisturized; (4) Dead surface cells that can cloud bright skin are eliminated . . . Exercise helps to lift and tighten the face and neck muscles so skin remains firmer and retains its elasticity. Facialistics care for your skin not only for today—but for the future as well."

In the Payot Skin Collections, there is the Noctis Series, consisting of a morning and night lotion, a light-textured night cream, and Masque Noctis, a zippy, peel-off mask; all of which are recommended for normal or sensitive, young skin that needs gentle care. The lotion, night cream, and mask, says Payot, "contain azulene, a soothing, natural extract of camomile and cytochromes which oxygenate the skin." In its Young & Problem Skin Series, Payot offers a total of six items, each "formulated to thoroughly cleanse, unclog pores, help clear up and guard against skin flare-ups, blemishes, and blackheads." Each product in Payot's Amnioderm Series contains amniotic fluid that purportedly keeps skin supple and young. This series is for women over thirty with sensitive skin, and sports a Masque

Amnioderm that Payot vows will make you say, "Away with wrinkles!" It is a remoisturizing, anti-dryness, creamy gel mask that is reputed to be a great line minimizer. It tones the skin and makes it feel supple all in less than twenty minutes. In this same series, Payot supplies a special super-rich Creme Amnioderm that guards against wrinkling even while you sleep. It is not patted on, but firmly massaged into the skin before bedtime. Also worth noting is Payot's Masque Hemera, which is a one-of-a-kind penetrating treatment, which is supposed to texturize the skin while minimizing lines, preventing dryness, and perking up tired skin. It can be used under makeup and reportedly helps subdue wrinkles when it is left on overnight.

It is always quite interesting when a cosmetics company centers its approach on completeness—something for everything and everybody—and when all the products bear the same company name, not a slew of subsidiaries turning out bright items with bright names. Payot markets so many skin products around the world that a buyer instantly gets the impression that "this company really knows all about skin conditions and whatever it has for those conditions must be good." No wonder Payot turns out its multi-purpose products in series. Payot's Classical Series, a bevy of cleansers and follow-up lotions and toners, are all designed to meet the needs of any type of skin. The advertising approach on some of the items is unique in its succinctness and directness: "Tired, puffy eyes? Soothe away the cares and reduce the puffs, even calm irritated eyelids, with this (Lotion Bleue) restful eye lotion." Also in the Payot Classical Series are numerous moisturizers and five night creams, each requiring massages, and all intended to banish lines from the face and neck. To top off the Payot difference is its Body Series—creams for the hands, legs, breasts, and abdominal area. Payot's cream will not remove "stretch" marks, but purportedly "discourages" them. The breast cream is admittedly a "novel" one, made with collagen, extracts of roses and citrus fruits, and certain moisturizers that help firm the breasts while nourishing them with moisture.

Payot is not a new cosmetics line, although most American women will immediately confess to knowing nothing about the products. Some say they have never heard of Payot at all. But Dr. Nadine G. Payot, a dermatologist and chemist, developed her skin-care program in France in 1919. Dedicated to helping women achieve and maintain healthy, beautiful skin, she also devised her Facialistics program, a unique and praised daily, at-home skin-care program.

It appears that most cosmetics companies today have tailored their products and selling techniques to that mass of women past thirty-five who, because of earlier skin neglect, are now in need of skin treatments. It probably goes without saying that women in this category created, although unintentionally, this great new (and still growing) market for cosmetics, albeit through faults and habits of their own. In a few years perhaps, most firms will have completely new skin-care cosmetics lines aimed at teenagers and those in their early twenties who ordinarily are concerned only with pimples and looking in style. Skin care is important even then because most skin damage begins in these early years. Good skin care can be advertised to be as much a treat as a new cheek blush.

Younger people *must* be impressed with the need for good nutrition, proper exercise, essential vitamins, and the proper care of their facial skin. Even Clearacil is a cosmetic treatment. Anyone using it must be taught not just what causes adolescent pimples, but what can be done to prevent them. Young women, and men, must be taught early the dangers of the sun, and how to counteract those dangers.

In a short time, a whole new world is going to open up for cosmetics, and especially for skin-treatment products. More and more stores will have to hire skin-care salespersons who can efficiently and helpfully assess the skin problems of customers and guide them safely and mercifully to products created for their conditions. People with skin conditions are coming out of the closets and openly seeking helpful information on what to do to alleviate their problems. Whether or not cosmetics stores ever do this, the health stores already are.

CHAPTER VII

MASQUES and MASSAGES: SOMETHING FROM THE PAST

My face shall wear a mask of care.

"Hunting Joy," Stanza 3

Facial masks, or masques, and packs are staging a very strong comeback, as are facial massages and exercises. Nobody seems to know why they went out of style, but for many years few cosmetics companies or beauty salons promoted them. Emphasis was placed instead on makeup techniques and hair styles.

There was a time, a number of years ago, when women relied on masks and packs as a facial cure-all— cleanser, toner, tension reliever, and wrinkle remover. The masks were made from everything: clay dirt, strawberries, buttermilk, watermelon juice (a good tightener), lemon juice, and even starch. Now they are back in force. Heavy attention is being given to herbal and fruit masks, and so-called peel-off packs. Flower masks are also coming on strong. And the biggest cosmetics companies now number high on their sales rosters specially formulated cosmetics for facial masks and packs. These, too, contain fruits, herbs, and hormones, not to mention a liberal assortment of vitamins.

THE WHYS, WHATS, AND HOWS OF FACIAL MASKS

Do Masks and Packs Do Any Good?

Proponents of facial masks and the thicker facial packs have said for years that they do shrink wrinkles, shrivel pores, cleanse, and relieve tension in face and neck muscles. Opponents, such as the American Medical Association, say masks and packs do the face and neck no substantial good. From my own experience, not just with my own skin but working with other people in an advisory capacity, I can say that facial masks and packs are, as a supplement, greatly helpful as a skin toner and cleanser. They surely invigorate the skin, and make a person feel alive and less tense. Masks and packs can loosen blackheads, making them disgorge from the skin and eventually push out on account of the skin's own eruptive action. And when they are used in conjunction with the other good skin-care suggestions mentioned in this book, they can help ban lines and wrinkles.

Why Did Women Stop Getting Facials?

Before the forties, women had a lot of time on their hands. Like the men of the sporting and leisure set, they could slip off to the beauty salon, and even to the barber salon, lie back in a reclining chair, and get their faces "worked on" professionally. Attendants would hot-towel their faces into receptive softness, apply astringents and cleansers, massage, rub, and squeeze. Out came the impurities, and the skin would spring into refreshed new life.

By the forties, women began to go to work by the millions. This increased in the fifties, and by the sixties, everything hit the fan. Women's Lib was upon us. Women, like men, found they had little or no time to spend in a beauty salon. They hurriedly bought makeup items, neglecting or forgetting the finer points of skin care. Cakes and coffee, sumptuous dinners, and exotic drinks became the vogue. So did bad skin. It is a fact that many women thrust suddenly into workaday life, who found they no longer had time to lie around getting facials in beauty salons, also found no time for such meticulous practices when they got home. The telephone, caring for the kids, social functions, and countless other things got in the way. The alarm bell did not ring loudly enough to be heard until mirrors began telling them that their makeup, bad diets, stress, insufficient rest and facial exercise, and too many hours in the sun had done them wrong.

Why The Revival of Clay Masks?

Women have been getting dirty faces for centuries using nature's oldest cleanser and healer, clay. Cleopatra used clay mud from the Nile on her face and body "to achieve smoothness of skin." Pliny the Elder wrote extensively in his *Natural History* of the helpful qualities of clay, and contemporary scientists attest to the special qualities of this mineral-rich natural product. But for years, women abstained from mudding up with clay dirt. Now clay is back, along with anything else that will help a troubled skin. Clay is non-toxic. In fact, some people actually drink clay mixed with water or fruit juice, regarding it as a helpful mineral tonic. It is popular in Europe in clay packs and masques for the skin. Clay is a natural deodorizer, and is highly absorbent. It can soak up excess oil and grime like a sponge.

142

It holds in moisture, and as it dries, it tightens the skin. Plus, it has a pH factor close to that of average skin. The rose clay from the quarries south of Paris are regarded as good for facial masks and packs. Pierre Cattier markets the *nature de France* rose clay worldwide in powder form, lotions, tonics, shampoos, conditioners, and even soaps, often found in health stores.

What About Home-Made Fruit Packs?

Antoine Marengo, formerly with the L'Oreal Company in France and with Elizabeth Arden, and who now lectures on skin care, said he felt American women generally laugh at putting juices and other foods on their faces. "Americans are too advanced to put food on their faces," he said. "With all that chemists have developed, we have evolved too far to stick egg or mayonnaise on our skin." But I feel that women today are concerned enough about skin conditions to try almost anything. If they can use clay dirt, why not certain food derivatives? True, we have facial packs especially mixed with fruit, herbs, and hormones, and they are a glory to use. But for those women who want their own thing, go to it. Kiehl's Pharmacy in New York City markets a Rare Earth Facial Cleansing Masque that contains rare clays, vitamin E, wheat germ, and avocado and peach oils. And Tove Borgnine (Mrs. Ernest Borgnine) offers her Tova 9 Collection in Beverly Hills and New York stores, which includes a masque made from cactus pulp, guaranteed to moisturize the driest face.

I also suggest an avocado mask made from a fully ripened avocado. A popular item for people who live in sunny climates and for a woman seeking to shrink enlarged pores and banish sallowness. First, mash half an avocado. Then, mix it into a paste with one tablespoon

143

of honey and one quarter of a cup of milk at room temperature. Blend thoroughly, apply to a clean face and neck, and leave on for thirty minutes. Remove with warm water, dab-drying lightly after patting on cold water.

Will Figs Help Bags Under the Eyes?

A lot of women have asked me this question. I don't know where they picked up the fig idea, but it registered with them. As a spot mask, figs are ideal for those dark circles under the eyes. The big problem is finding a store that sells fresh figs. If you are lucky enough to find them, take two of them, crush or slice them open, place one part over each eye lid and one part under each eye while lying down. Stay reclined for twenty or thirty minutes, remove the fruit parts, and dab clean with a moistured towelette. Do this daily for about two weeks and sing praises of the results.

What About The Rest of the Face?

Let's try the "natural" pack first. Cleanse the face and neck with a mild soap, like Neutrogena. Get yourself some fennel leaves (an aromatic herb in the parsley family). Make a tea with a tablespoonful of the leaves and water. Then mix equal parts of the tea with equal portions of yogurt and honey. Apply the paste to lined and wrinkled areas of the face and neck, taking care not to pack around the eyes. After reclining with the pack for half an hour, wash off with lukewarm, soapless water, and pat the skin lightly dry. A bit of honey rubbed around the eyes nightly will help those areas. After a month of this daily regimen, you should see some real smoothing results.

For similarly aging skin conditions, there are some

highly respected cosmetics that achieve good results when applied as masks and packs. Lancôme's Mask No. 10 is a clear gel hydrating mask. It's made from seaweed and sea-water extracts. It reduces puffiness under the eyes, and hydrates and firms the skin. It is a quick, refreshing pickup. Payot has two masks for lines and wrinkles, the Masque Amnioderm and the Masque Hemera. The one from the Amnioderm Series challenges wrinkles to the utmost. It is a remoisturizing, anti-dryness, creamy gel mask that helps minimize fine lines. It tones and supples skin in fifteen to twenty minutes. The Masque Hemera is a one-of-a-kind penetrating mask designed to give the skin texture while also helping to diminish fine lines. When left on overnight, it perks up tired skin and helps subdue wrinkles. Hemera, applied thinly, can be left to dry and then used under makeup as an all-day mask.

Should Masks Be Used Daily?

Not really. For extreme skin conditions, daily applications are recommended for at least two weeks, whether you use a natural or a chemically formulated mixture. Later on, apply only two or three times weekly for a month. Not only are various ingredients in masks used for toning, but they are also used for getting rid of wrinkles and crow's-feet.

Specifically, What Do Certain Natural Products Do?

We are all products of Mother Earth, and whether the ingredients in your mask come from the garden or the cosmetics counter, you are bound to be using something from the soil or ocean. A book the size of a Sears catalogue could not describe all the earth-derived products that could be used to heal, help, or harm the skin. But let's take a very few commonly known items. *Lemon juice*: bleaches, tightens, shrinks pores, and reduces alkalinity. A citric acid, it is the acid most often used in cosmetics. Lime juice has the same qualities only more so; both can be irritating. *Strawberries*: soften and nourish the skin. *Raspberries*: the juice is a perky astringent. *Honey*: softens, nourishes, and bleaches the skin. People allergic to pollen should avoid items containing honey. *Eggs*: beaten egg whites, or the yolk alone, have been used in and for facial masks for many years. The albumin from eggs tightens facial skin, and puckers, or plumps it. *Oatmeal*: uncooked and mixed with warm water and patted on the face and neck, it works well as a poultice, drawing embedded impurities to the surface. (Do not use too often.) *Meal*: (corn or almond) a mask from either of these meals is beneficial. A paste made from almond meal and water, left on the face for about fifteen minutes, is splendid for refining the skin, removing blackheads, and diminishing large pores. Oatmeal has been considered a good skin cleansing agent for a long time. It is high in minerals and vitamins. Oatmeal soap was popular in Grandma's day.

If Natural Masks Are Good, Why Use Cosmetics?

Again, to each his or her own. Some people eat no meat. Some people prefer natural to synthetic vitamins. Some people think *all* cosmetics that are not all-natural are harmful and even sinful, even though some synthetic products are more powerful than natural ones. Everybody seeks to be on the *only* side, completely for this and completely against that, as if there is one perfect solution. Counter cosmetics today mix and blend ingredients from all kinds of sources, and with beneficial results. But no single cosmetic, natural or synthetic, will prevent or remove lines and wrinkles, or prevent aging. Help *must* come from a combination of sources. Persons can be allergic to certain natural herbs, fruits, flowers, and vegetables, just as they can be allergic to certain chemicals in counter cosmetics. No one thing is magical. It is true that what we use on our faces is a factor in how our skin looks, but so is what we eat. Alcoholic beverages and smoking can ruin the world's greatest skin-care regimen. Persons who drink heavily show it in their faces, and also show improvements when they let up. Skin invariably clears when heavy smokers let up or stop. Stress and constant nervousness make any skin dilate and erupt in pimples and lines. Selective vitamins, especially if they are used at certain ages, are good for maintaining a healthful, smooth skin if other conditions are favorable. And daily exercise of the skin should surely be added to the other favorable conditions.

Will Use of a Live-Cell Mask Make Me Grow Facial Hair?

No more than an egg-yolk mask will make you grow feathers. This is a question sometimes asked about the La Prairie facial mask that is enriched with preserved live-cell extracts of collagen, black-sheep placenta, and elastin. The La Prairie Masque is a good one. Its rich placental extract, collagen, and essential oils form an active, non-drying mask that aids dramatically in beautifying skin tissue. The mask should be applied to the face and throat, avoiding the areas around the eyes. Allow it to remain on the skin for about thirty minutes. It can then be tissued or rinsed off with lukewarm water. Use about twice weekly. La Prairie suggests that you use a gentle facial application of La Prairie Night Cream after the masque. For the neck areas, La Prairie offers its Cellular Neck Treatment, which contains elastin.

Should Soap or Cosmetics Cleansers Be Used Before Masking?

A universally good question. Soap should not be used to wash off makeup. Soap embeds makeup into the pores, enlarging them, whereas cleansers dissolve makeup. Cleansers often contain oil that's resistant to water moisture, however. An astringent or skin freshener would be best if you are not allergic to alcohol. Astringents contain about 0.4 percent alcohol, and are good for oily skin. Fresheners contain about 0.1 percent alcohol and are good for dry skin. Nearly all people have either oily or dry skin.

Do Moisturizers Work Better After Masking?

That depends on the type of mask being used. First, masks should not be used in lieu of gentle scrubbing or the natural course of skin exfoliation, which happens every twenty-eight days. There is generally some dead, flaky skin lying on top of the epidermis at all times, slowly but steadily peeling off to allow the regeneration of a new protective layer of skin. Clothing most often rubs off the flaking skin on our bodies. But on our faces and the upper part of our necks, we must use the rubbing process. Peeling, some call it. Some do it too much, trying always to find a new skin layer. Ordinary soaps usually scour off this skin. Their strong alkalis flush away surface acids and make the skin dry and brittle. Strong soaps harm delicate new skin. Some women use Noxema Medicated Skin Cream to "slough off those dead drab cells," rinsing afterwards with warm

148

water and patting dry. If you go in for soap, try to find a brand formulated from amino acids extracted from milk. Moisturizers work best after cleansing, not necessarily after masking.

Should Facial Tissues or Towels Be Used for Facial Scrubbing?

Too much scrubbing endangers growing skin. Few faces require actual scrubbing. Drying, yes; scrubbing, no. But if scrub you must, do it gently by mostly blotting. Facial tissues are usually made from wood pulp, and towels and wash cloths are made from synthetic and cotton fibers, sometimes silk. But you should find your best friend in cottonballs and cosmetic washcloths. They wash out easily and cost about six dollars for a package of six.

What's to a Photo-Facial?

Nothing more than a chance for you to get a visual imprint of the lines, wrinkles and pimples on your face. Max Factor's Geminesse line created the Photo Facial Moisture Mask. Marketed as a complete facial treatment, you begin by using the Conditioning Primer, which must dry before you apply the mask. Aside from providing the face with a refreshing feeling and cleansing it, the mask, when peeled off, gives you a photoprint of your skin, letting you see the trouble spots your skin has.

Do Scrub Masks Do Anything Besides Cleanse?

Not really. Once again, a mask generally freshens, stimulates, tones, refines, and cleanses your skin. A scrub mask may do a little more. Charles Revson's Ultima II Skim Milk Deep Pore Scrub Masque is a double-action pore cleanser. It is a combination of clay and scrub cream with natural almond grains. The clay draws out deep-down debris and excess oils during the twenty minutes it's on the skin. After the mask has dried, you must apply a few drops of water to the nose, forehead, and chin—the oiliest areas of the face. A few minutes of gentle scrubbing whisks off dead skin. Finish with a lukewarm water rinse.

Do Peel-Off Masks Hurt Coming Off?

Some of them do. After all, anything allowed to dry and harden on the skin is apt to sting when it is stripped off, but the sting is only momentary. A good peel-off mask, which starts with a lotion or cream, peels off in one continuous sheet, as Helena Rubinstein's Brush-on-Peel-Off Astringent Mask does. It would be good to follow the peeling with your favorite moisturizing lotion or cream, but even resilient peel-off masks pull the skin when they come off.

Is Dermabrasion Better Than Masks for Peeling?

Again, masks should not be considered a vehicle for skin peeling. If you feel that constantly shaving away at those surface skin conditions will in time give you a *new* face, forget it. I repeat, conditions are helped from within and without. Even cosmetic surgeons will tell you that they can do nothing about the chemical rebuilding factors within your body and beneath your skin that make for certain surface appearances, and they are experts at that peel-off business. But store-bought abrasives come in three varieties: the once-a-week rougher, the three-times-a-week semi-abrasive, and the non-abrasive peeler that can be used daily. Even after that, you must find and select a good neutralizer, a protein-fortified lotion, and then a good moisturizer. For ideal skin exfoliation, you may use Germaine Monteil's Facial Sluffing Cream, which is a safe and gentle exfoliating, or peeling, cream that helps brighten and polish the skin. It is a treatment that refines the skin's texture and stimulates surface circulation, and it is especially helpful in clearing troubled skin.

Do Skin-Tightening Masks Tone the Skin?

A toner is either an astringent or a skin freshener. It does not stimulate suppleness, elasticity, or firmness. Some women with saggy skin have, unfortunately, been led to believe that facial masks that dry on the skin, forming a tight mask like plaster of paris, firm up, supple, and "tone" the skin. Not so. Some are told that to try to move the facial muscles while this tightjacket is on the skin actually helps "tone" those muscles. Not so. If anything, such masks and such muscular movements under those masks can harm not only the muscles but the surface skin. Years ago, a product was introduced called Linit, a box of starch-like stuff, which, when mixed into a paste and applied like a mask to the face, dried into a viselike covering. People liked to try to smile or grimace while they were wearing it. Thankfully, it soon diminished in popularity. Again, masks are, according to Germaine Monteil, makers of the Clarity Color Timed Masque, to be used "to poultice and purge the complexion of impurities." They do invigorate, too, and at the most can make lines and wrinkles easier to deal with.

151

Is PABA Ever Used in Masks?

Yes, for one, Marian Bialac's PABA Treatment Masque, a pleasantly scented substance that dries and tightens the skin while the mask is on. Most masks and packs, however, do not dry or tighten, with PABA or without.

THE IMPORTANCE OF REGULAR FACIAL EXERCISE

Dr. M. J. (Joe) Saffon calls it the "Hollywood instant face lift." In his Prentice-Hall book, *The 15-Minute-A-Day Natural Face Lift,* and in a *Family Circle* magazine article and a *Midnight/Globe* diagrammed tableau, author Saffon described his facial exercise theories as the "no-surgery face lift." Saffon should know a lot about skin, since he worked at one time with Dr. Paul Niehans, founder of the La Prairie Clinic in Switzerland, and Saffon's father was a plastic surgeon. But all in all, what Saffon does promote, and quite successfully, is exercise of the facial muscles, something nobody had been pushing, except for Helena Rubinstein, for a number of years. It had been thought for a long time, and God knows who foisted this theory upon the public, that daily facial exercises would make the skin loose and saggy, that it would cause baggy eyes and even cause lines and wrinkles. Some women were afraid to smile too much for fear that it would cause the foregoing conditions. Cosmetics people didn't help straighten out this misconception, either, except for the Payot people who stressed facial exercises and skin massaging along with use of their cosmetics. La Prairie urged facial exercises, but at that time, La Prairie offered its live-cell therapy only by injection and only in Geneva at the famed clinic. The La Prairie cosmetics line had not yet been placed on the public market.

Physicians, who generally discredited all cosmetics, have never stopped urging people to do regular exercise of the facial and neck muscles as an aid to good skin health.

Dr. J. Frank Hurdle, in his book *Common Sense Health Manual* (Parker Publishing Co., Inc., 1975), says:

"There are four main sources of too many wrinkles and leather skin: the sun, the wind, excess fatty tissure, and the lack of facial muscle tone. . . . Losing weight down to ideal levels will automatically take off facial flab. It won't just hang there in folds *if you do proper toning of the facial muscles at the same time.* I've recently heard some plastic surgeons decry facial exercises as causing more wrinkles—as not being good for your face. I disagree."

Although Dr. Hurdle has not praised the introduction of hormones into the skin from outside the body, such as through the application of certain cosmetics, he does say that "physical tone *increases* total hormone production and causes these potent messengers to *stabilize* your body's defenses against infectious disease, stress, wear and tear on joints and muscles, breakdown of cells, aging, and ill health."

Why not just take hormones with a glass of water? Why not, for muscle tone, aging signs, and cell breakdowns just buy some counter cosmetics or use some home-made product on the skin for that deep-down penetration that gets the hormones into the body? Why exercise? Hurdle says that ingesting hormonal substances and applying them on the body isn't enough. He says, "The construction of our bodies isn't so simple, for every time one hormone is increased, one or more

153

other hormones have to be reduced. And maintaining this ever changing balance of hormones can only come as a result of their *natural* production right in your own body."

A lack of exercise *can* cause laziness and even stagnation of our skin cells. When exercise fires up these cells, they function a lot better and have a renewed and youthful vigor. Take skin-help vitamins and use cosmetics for your personal skin type and you are on the way to glowing skin beauty, he says. In fact, Dr. Hurdle adds rather profoundly that "physical toning and nutrition are inseparable partners in total health."

Romana de Vries, in her 1979 book *Cosmetrics* (E. P. Dutton), tells and shows why she is called "Hollywood's Face Magician," as she devotes virtually her entire book to photographs showing how to do facial exercises to attain "the natural way to a forever-young face." Miss de Vries contends, and quite rightly, that "elasticity of skin is determined by the strength and tone of the muscles," and that " improper use of these facial muscles creates wrinkles." The *Cosmetrics* author, who appears at times on television giving beauty tips, models in her own book. Her face has a few lines that could probably be helped by some of the new and helpful cosmetics products now on the market, but her skin shows a glowing vigor that undoubtedly was aided by a religious regimen of facial exercise.

What Exercises Should Be Used for Eye Areas?

The areas around the eyes reflect our diets and living habits more than they do our age. Saffon maintains that the areas around the eyes are the only area of the face that won't respond to his instant face-lift exercises, explaining as he did to Linda Konner of *US* magazine, "I can't help a person who already has bags or 'suitcases' under the eyes. Those can only be removed surgically."

That reminded me of my friend who has had four operations for bags under her eyes. In her case, I feel it is a genetic problem, having nothing to do with aging, diet, living habits, the sun, wind, or use of bad cosmetics, and surely nothing to do with lack of facial exercise. She developed bags under her eyes at the age of twenty.

But Dr. J. Frank Hurdle explains that "bags beneath the eyes mean that your health control needs boosting. The skin beneath your eyes is rather thin anyway, and if the muscle beneath this skin—a circular muscle that surrounds the entire eye—is lax, fluid normally present in the tissues collects in abundance and puffs the skin out. The eye exercise is done by forcibly closing your eyes and with pressure, alternately contracting and relaxing this circular muscle. A finger placed below your eye will tell you if you're doing this correctly—you can feel the circular muscle bunch up."

Hurdle recommends that this exercise be performed for five minutes each day, followed by a massage of the areas around the eyes with a selected skin lotion or facial cream. He also suggests that you place an ice cube on the pouch sector for five minutes before applying the cosmetics. Earlier in this book, I outlined an eye exercise similar to the one suggested by Dr. Hurdle, and I know it works. But I know also, in agreement with the Payot eye-exercise formula, that the delicate and thin skin around the eyes should not be stretched or pulled. Puffiness has already stretched it. You want it to contract, lineless, as exercise, diet, and moisturization get the puffiness underneath that light outer skin to subside, or contract.

If the area around your eyes is merely lined, a good

regimen of vitamin C with its collagen-making abilities, in combination with vitamin P (bioflavonoids), along with any of the good eye-area cosmetics listed in this book, will help. Don't forget fig masks for dark circles under the eyes.

The muscles of the eyes can be toned by gently pressing two fingers on each side of your head, directly at the temples, and opening and closing your eyes with gusto several times each day.

What Is an Exercise for Chins Tending to Double?

There are several, some vigorous, others more gentle. I, like many other cosmetics counselors, suggest the gentle one introduced some years back by the late Helena Rubinstein. Place the back of your hand beneath the chin, push upward and backward with your hand while pushing forward and downward with your chin and simultaneously contracting the neck muscles.

For a more strenous chin exercise, one practiced by prizefighters, simply drop the chin down on the chest while contracting the neck muscles back and forth vigorously. And while you are at it, give the neck muscles a good daily workout by tilting the head around and back and forth while contracting the neck muscles. Also place a hand firmly at the nape of the neck while tossing your head back several times against the firm hand.

Are There Exercises for the Mouth and Cheeks?

And how! It's better if they are begun early in life and kept up over the years. But in case your face has been living a sedentary life along with your body as "tired" conditions developed, this little series of face joggers should help: Remember that people who whistle a lot seldom have lines around the mouth. Whistle

156

while you work, while you cook, and anytime you can, even if you don't make a sound. Just act like you are whistling, pursing your lips over your teeth and hold them there for several minutes while holding your mouth open as wide as you can. Smile without puckering your lips. You can also purse your lips and swing your mouth from side to side; this also strengthens cheek muscles. Make like you are saying "ooh." This is one of the oldest mouth exercises, and it's done most effectively while you hold your hands firmly on each side of your lower face while pushing upward. After a daily go at these exercises, cleanse your face thoroughly and apply a good protein-fortified emollient, then a good penetrating moisturizer.

Should Lotions Ever be Applied Before Exercising?

If your skin is very dry, by all means use a good hand lotion, like Vaseline's Intensive Care, or a cold cream on the areas to be massaged. Afterward, cleanse them off and rub in your moisturizer.

Are Isometrics Any Good for the Face?

Isometrics (tensing one set of mucles against an immoble set) are ideal for the face if you don't mind grimacing like a clown often during the day. You should try it, as it's highly beneficial. For instance, if, when you rise in the morning, you try to touch your nose with your tongue, you will feel your face muscles getting one of the best exercises possible. Don't feel silly trying it. You should have tried it years ago. It is one of the best neck, chin, and cheek workouts, and it also stimulates the upper muscles on each side of the face. You can also tense your nose and cheek muscles isometrically. And bully for you if you can wiggle your ears!

Do the Lips Need Any Exercise?

Yes, they do, and generally they get a lot of exercise during the day as we talk, drink, eat, smoke, smile, and pucker. But they can benefit from isometric pursing and puckering during idle moments. Don't forget that the lips need special pampering to remain soft and attractive. Whenever you are treating your face, apply a liberal amount of moisturizing cream or lotion to your lips. It will provide a superb base for a longer-lasting and more natural-looking application of lipstick, and it prevents peeling and chapping.

What's Good for the Chin, Forehead and Nose?

Around the forehead, there is what anatomists call the temporalis muscle, which usually gets little regular exercise. The muscle is at the upper part of each side of your face. When it's tired, your jowls are apt to sag. Spruce up this muscle daily by placing your palms against it, at each temple, and moving the palms around in a circle while holding the jaw closed tight and pressing the fingers toward the center of the forehead. The muscle at the center of the forehead can be exercised by using two fingers of each hand to press alternately up and down several times daily on it, back and forth across the forehead. This action stimulates circulation and muscle tone. And the same two fingers should be used similarly, with up and down motions, pressing directly between the eyebrows, to iron out those frown lines.

As to the frontal part of the chin and the lines on it, simply tuck your top lip down into your mouth, covering it as much as possible with your bottom lip. This action will make it feel like your chin is thrusting out. It is. Hold the position steady for about half a minute, or for as long as you can. Do this each morning and at night.

The area around the nose is very sensitive. Pressing on the area adjacent to the nose sometimes brings on sneezes and/or sinus discomfort. But that area, and the nose itself, should get some exercise. The wings of the nose should be massaged with the middle finger, by using circular motions for about thirty seconds and then gently sliding the finger upward several times to the bridge of the nose. Using the forefinger and the thumb, lightly pinch the tip of the nose, tilting the tip from side to side until it feels more alive.

Can't Facial Massages Save You All This Work?

Getting someone else to do these facial and neck exercises for you would save you some energy, but it would surely not save you money. Whereas twenty years ago, a facial in a salon could cost from three to ten dollars, the same work today could cost up to a hundred dollars. And you need to do these exercises daily. But if you have a beauty expert, male or female, who could give you a bargain facial massage two or three times a week and if you can fit it into your budget, you are almost home free. A member of your family could do it, following the directions in this book, as some women cannot press with their fingers or hands too firmly because of problems such as arthritis.

Barbers, who have watched their hair-cutting business move "uptown," are usually good at giving facial massages. They could also offer bargains, to the woman who does not want to do the facials herself.

Most women can do these facial gymnastics themselves, and enjoy doing it. And their enthusiasm will grow as they feel and see the results. Any woman using cosmetics today should change her pat-on routine to one of massaging in some of the substances, which not only helps the cosmetic to work into the skin better, but also helps stimulate and invigorate the skin muscles underneath.

Many shops in many cities now advertise the so-called non-surgical face lift. But keep in mind, you can give yourself a daily lift without cost.

Lida Livingston and Constance Schrader's book *Wrinkles, How to Prevent Them, How to Erase Them* (Prentice-Hall), in general, suggests the facial exercises described in this book, but also suggests that they be done with moisturizers, olive or vegetable oil, or safflower mayonnaise applied to the face, followed by an application of heated spoons around the lined and wrinkled facial areas. The book was heralded in the *National Enquirer* as the way: "you can iron away your wrinkles at home using an amazingly simple technique."

What About Ginseng Tea for the Skin?

Ginseng has been recommended for everything. It is touted as a sexual stimulant. I know some skin cosmetics have ginseng in them, but I have yet to be shown how it does the skin any good. It purportedly regulates menstrual periods and could possibly help control skin problems related to menstruation. Ginseng does perk up glands and awaken the nervous system. It grows commercially in the United States, although people who use it prefer the Korean root and especially the one that looks somewhat like a human torso. Movie actress Sharon Farrell told beauty columnist Lydia Lane that Ginseng tea bags brewed in hot water relieved her puffy eyelids and improved her hair, nails, and skin. The Chinese claim it helps you live longer, and judging from China's populations, who can argue?

160

CHAPTER VIII
VITAMINS AND DIETS FOR A YOUTHFUL SKIN

There are two things every woman prays for. One is a flawless skin. The other is a healthy, slender body.

Helena Rubinstein

I am still looking for that woman who is lucky enough to have flawless skin. I have known many with healthy, slender bodies. But every one of them was actively engaged in the hot pursuit of a youthful complexion and postponing any sign of aging.

Aside from the attractive appearance certain cosmetics afford you, the increased circulation stimulated by facial exercise, the smoothness and glow of a sun-sheltered skin, the clean feeling provided by facial masks and packs, those factors most often having to do with a healthy, youthful skin have long been due to adequate intake of the right vitamins.

Many skin changes having to do with aging are caused by deficiencies in certain vitamins. Pimples and blackheads and a pallid complexion, not to mention collagen breakdown, may be caused by a chronic lack of certain vitamins, too.

Some women with dry skin nightly cleanse, tone, and massage all-night moisturizers into their skin only to find that their problem remains the same. But, after increasing their intake of vitamin A, they note changes for the better. The help the body is getting from within helps the cosmetics do what is expected of them.

Research has shown that whether you use synthetic or natural cosmetics your skin health is most assured if you have the right diet and take the right vitamins. Most of us eat a lot, but generally we do not eat the right foods. We take vitamins, but generally our bodies lack certain vitamins necessary to good skin health. And at certain ages, our bodies undergo changes requiring increased amounts of certain vitamins. In some cases, a deficiency in one vitamin will cause us to stop manufacturing other vital vitamins necessary to the production of cell-building protein. Some beauty experts have for a long time urged that we stop drinking water, and have suggested that juices or the water in fruits will suffice. Large amounts of water are a must daily for anybody who wants to have healthy skin. Anyone suffering from a lack of carbohydrates will be even worse off if he or she does not drink enough water. And without water and carbohydrates, the kidneys are unable to metabolize fats.

Sure, exercise helps, no matter what your age, but you will not be able to exercise regularly if you have an inadequate supply of vitamins and the proper foods.

You can fast and rest, sleep your life away, seeking a clear complexion, but even a slow-moving and sedentary body requires vitamins and a proper diet. Vitamins help your body use the food you eat to give you energy and keep you and your skin healthy. Every cell in your body needs vitamins to function. Minerals, the great regulators, also help the body run well, assisting facial muscles, giving nerves a boost, and keeping the water balance in the body.

From the childhood on, most Americans are locked

into a pattern whereby they do not get the minimum daily requirements of vitamins. This is due mainly to unbalanced diets and eating patterns that provide too much of one or two vitamins and little or none of the necessary vitamins. Few children get all the nutrients their growing bodies need, especially iron and vitamins A and C. And the results become compounded when they stop growing, in their twenties, and "aging" starts a reverse cycle.

Adults who are heavy smokers lose large amounts of vitamin C, and steady drinking can lead to an improper utilization of vitamins B-1 and B-6 and folic acid—all of which are related to skin health. Some women who are taking oral contraceptives suffer from skin eruptions during their periods. They often need an extra supply of vitamins B-1, B-2, B-12, C, and folic acid.

If a younger-looking face is your objective, do not overlook the importance of certain skin-vitalizing vitamins. A lack of fatty acids in the body can produce skin disorders, but an excessive amount of fat in the diet can lead to obesity, among other things. Four or five tablespoons of unsaturated vegetable oil mixed into your food daily will do wonders for your skin. Protein and water are directly responsible for the health of the muscles and skin. Protein also helps maintain a proper acid balance. Proteins form enzymes that are necessary if antibodies are going to fight off skin infections and skin "tiredness." Protein is the major building material for the body.

Vegetables that supply amino acids help the body build proteins. To do this, they must supply eight amino acids that combine with fourteen other amino acids in a specific pattern to make protein. Animo acids actually synthesize body proteins and the components of skin tissue. All twenty-two amino acids must be present in their natural order and proportion, at the same time, to

163

produce this protein synthesis. Some foods provide *complete protein* factors; other foods, like vegetables, provide *incomplete protein* factors, causing a need for vitamin supplements.

How Much Protein Do We Need Daily?

Dr. Charles S. Davidson, M.D., of Harvard Medical School, claims that skin wrinkles are caused by a deficiency in protein. And I recall reading in a magazine article that skin aging can be warded off by ingesting 126 grams of protein daily, a contention to which I could not readily subscribe. Some women supplement their daily diets by drinking a glass of fruit juice with two or three tablespoons of powdered protein in it. But if you weigh 120 pounds, your body requires 60 grams of protein daily. An easy way to figure your daily protein need is to follow the National Research Council's guide of 0.42 grams daily for each pound you weigh. Divide your weight by two, and you get the number of grams of protein you should have each day. Of course, to prevent protein deficiency, you *can* ingest more than is needed. Stress and illness can cause your body to lose protein. You're probably best off if your daily diet is low on calories and high in proteins, but try to avoid becoming engulfed in a "protein mystique." Too much of anything can be bad. A welcome balance could be obtained easily if we would follow early-American basic menus that included brown rice, barley, oatmeal, wheat, bran, assortments of ripe fruits, peas, beans, carrots, raw vegetables, and slightly cooked green-leaf and yellow vegetables; yams (with no refined sugar added), corn, squash, eggplant, and a few small portions daily of lean meat for a supply of B-12, for those who are not already taking B-12 vitamins.

Care and Feeding of the Skin from Within

A healthy skin must be well fed from within and without. An oily skin may reflect a deficiency of vitamin B-2, or riboflavin, which can be obtained from milk or liver, among other foods. An oily skin beset with pimples can be caused by a lack of vitamin B-6, or pyridoxine, found in bananas, wheat germ, pork and veal, fish (salmon, sardines), yellow corn, milk, soybeans and rice, and whole-grain bread. Pyridoxine (B-6) helps the body use B-12, and as a coenzyme helps the body make use of carbohydrates, fats, and proteins. You can't build red blood cells without it. It also converts the essential amino acid tryptophan to niacin, and synthesizes and activates DNA and RNA. The body does not store pyridoxine. After it has been in the body for about half a day, it is excreted through the urine. If you go on a fast, pyridoxine is eliminated from your body very quickly. Adults need at least 2 milligrams per 100 grams of protein per day.

Doctors say women taking birth-control pills lose large amounts of vitamin B-6 and folic acid. It is always safe to assume that any skin showing premature signs of aging reflects a body suffering from a lack of sufficient B-complex vitamins.

Vitamin A, Friend of the Skin

Without a doubt, the vitamin for the skin is vitamin A, the fat-soluble nutrient vital to growth and repair of body tissues. It stimulates production of smooth, soft skin. It fights off infection, builds strong bones, durable teeth, and good eyesight. It is great for the treatment of facial and other skin blemishes, pimples, warts, acne, and rashes—from the outside. On the inside, it fights

165

stress ulcers, asthma, pre-menstrual symptoms—any conditions that are liable to be manifested on the skin. Aside from the 10,000 IU capsules of synthetic and natural vitamin A found almost everywhere, you can get vitamin A from fish-liver oils, in cream and butter, in carrots, beets, squash, broccoli, and dark-green and deep-gold vegetables. Carrots supply carotene, which the body converts into vitamin A. Without sufficient A, the body devours any vitamin C that is in the body. Daily ingestions of magnesium and vitamin A aid skin moisturization.

IMPORTANT SKIN-HELP VITAMINS

Americans spend $500 million yearly on water-soluble and fat-soluble vitamins. The water-soluble vitamins—C, "bioflavonoids," and the B-complex—are measured in milligrams. Fat-soluble vitamins—A, D, E, F and K— are measured in "International Units," or IU's. RDA means Recommended Daily Allowance for adults.

VITAMIN A (Retinol)

RDA 10,000 IU. A fat-soluble vitamin that accumulates in the body; it is used in many cosmetics for its proven skin-healing abilities. It can be absorbed through the skin. A vitamins are necessary for new cell growth. Vitamin A aids the functioning of our eyes, skin, teeth, guns, and mucous membranes; it attacks acne, skin cancers, and protects against air pollutants. Ten thousand or 25,000 International Units daily are alright, although some people take a total of 50,000 IU's daily. Extra-high amounts of vitamin A can be dangerous to your health. I found this out the hard way.

In those days before there was a maximum of 10,000 IU's in vitamin A capsules sold over the counter, I was taking several 25,000 IU vitamin A capsules daily to ward off skin eruptions brought on not only by menstrual periods but by birth-control pills. After a time, I began to suffer terribly painful headaches every night. My menstrual periods became erratic, and my face began erupting in tiny volcanoes. My doctors didn't know what was causing this. But as soon as it was announced in the newspapers that vitamin A in large dosages could bring on such symptoms, and could create cellular damage, I stopped taking more than 10,000 IU's daily. My symptoms disappeared and have never come back.

VITAMIN B-1 (Thiamine)

RDA 1.5 milligrams. Water-soluble. Increases metabolism of sugars for energy, improves muscle tone, sharpens the mind, and fights Herpes. It is found in wheat, bran, molasses, rice, corn, ham, liver, pork roasts, grapefruit, nuts, asparagus, greens, avocados, and lima beans, most of which are also very high in proteins.

VITAMIN B-2 (Riboflavin)

RDA 1.2 for females, 1.6 for males. Water-soluble. It is in liver, tongue, and other organ meats, eggs, milk, and nuts, dark poultry meat, and most of all in brewer's yeast, many foods that also provide B-1. Riboflavin helps other enzymes break up and use carbohydrates, fats, and proteins. It is necessary for the maintenance of good skin. Alcohol uses up the body's B-2. Restricted diets for the treatment of ulcers and diabetes are also dangerous to the body's B-2.

VITAMIN B-3 (Niacin)

About 16 milligrams recommended daily. Water-soluble. Niacin aids energy production in cells, strengthens muscles, prevents rough skin, skin inflammation, depression, and bad breath. It works best when and if it is taken in the entire B-complex combination. It is found in brewer's yeast, tuna, peanuts, white enriched bread (and other wheat and rye breads), in liver, mushrooms, and white poultry meat.

VITAMIN B-6 (Pyridoxine)

RDA 2 milligrams for each 100 grams of protein. B-6 should always be taken as part of the whole B-complex line, never alone, since it works best in combination with the other B vitamins. These B vitamins prompt the liver to make glycogen, which helps the skin exfoliate, or cast off, dead skin cells. They help the body offset damages caused by stress, depression, too much coffee, and too much alcohol.

BIOTIN

RDA 100 to 300 micrograms daily. Water-soluble. Biotin, a B-complex vitamin, prevents scaling dermatitis. A coenzyme that makes fatty acids and aids in the body's use of folic acid, protein, B-12, and pantothenic acid. Liver, peanuts, brewer's yeast, eggs, and dried beans abound in biotin.

PANTOTHENIC ACID

Suggested daily need; 5 to 50 milligrams. It is a B-complex vitamin found in all living cells—eggs, meats,

168

yeast, and whole-grain cereals. Aids in cell metabolism and the production of hormones necessary for healthy skin. It utilizes energy from fats and proteins. It is a proven aid in the prevention of wrinkles, and protects skin cells from getting damaged by the sun.

INOSITOL

RDA 100 to 300 milligrams daily. It helps the body manufacture lecithin to remove fats from the liver. It prevents hair from falling out. It is found in citrus fruits, yeast, liver, and molasses. Coffee is an enemy of inositol.

CHOLINE

RDA 1,000 milligrams. People suffering from heart conditions are often given more choline, since it is regarded as the great emulsifier, in that it dissolves and emulsifies cholesterol in the bloodstream so that it won't settle on arterial walls. It protects the liver from alcohol, too. If you are a drinker, you should also take larger supplements of choline. It is an ingredient of lecithin. It is great for nerves, strengthens weak capillaries, cleans eyes, and fights eczema. Food rich in choline are eggs, poultry, fish, beef, pork, leafy vegetables, wheat bran, wheat germ, and brewer's yeast. If you have heard that eggs are rich in cholesterol, please be advised that eggs are also rich in choline, which renders cholesterol harmless in the arteries.

VITAMIN B-12

RDA 3 to 5 milligrams daily. Water-soluble. It is the most powerful vitamin. It contains cobalt and phosphorus. It is available in low-priced tablet form, and in higher dosages for persons who may have pernicious anemia. Many vegetarians suffer from a lack of B-12, for it exists almost exclusively in animal meat, fish, and milk. It is also found in yeast, soybeans, and wheat germ. Vitamin B-12 is essential for longevity, being the only vitamin with essential mineral elements. It fights psoriasis and shingles. A deficiency can cause a persistent body odor.

VITAMIN B-13 (Orotic Acid)

This B vitamin is available only outside the United States. A deficiency in this vitamin can cause dry skin, cell degeneration, and premature aging. In the body, B-13 metabolizes B-12 and folic acid. Research in Russia and West Germany has proven that orotic acid can restore skin cells.

PABA (Para-amino-benzoic Acid)

RDA 30 milligrams. Water-soluble. PABA is a B-complex vitamin that works in direct combination with folic acid. It makes intestinal bacteria produce folic acid, which in turn helps produce pantothenic acid. The body also makes its own PABA, but apparently not enough. Sulfa drugs hamper PABA's effectiveness. It is good for treating burns, skin discolorations, and for preventing sunburn. PABA also effectively retards skin changes caused by aging, and combats dry skin. It is available in tablet form, and is found in foods such as yogurt, liver, wheat germ, and molasses. PABA is also an ingredient in most of the sun screens and sun-block cosmetics on the market, and is in numerous cosmetics designed to combat aging skin.

FOLIC ACID

RDA 400 mcg. Water-soluble. Part of the B-complex. A coenzyme, it works with B-12 and vitamin C in the body to break down and utilize proteins. It builds red blood cells, and forms nucleic acid, essential for growth and reproduction of all body cells, including those of the facial skin. Stress, sickness, and alcoholism make it more difficult for the body to produce folic acid. It is found in tablet form at vitamin counters and in foods such as beef, pork, fish, poultry, vegetables, fruits, cheeses, milk, eggs, whole grain cereals, tree and bush nuts, and in ground-seed items such as soybeans, peanuts, and sunflower seeds. Liver is abundant with it, which is why some people sprinkle desiccated liver on salads.

VITAMIN B-15 (Pangamic Acid)

This vitamin, part of the vitamin B-complex, is called the "banned" vitamin, since it is always being forced off health and vitamin store shelves because authorities say it has no proven value. For many years, authorities said the same thing about vitamin E.

One thing worth noting is that medical authorities who are forcing some presumably "no help" product from the market are always more forceful than they are when they are taking harmful products from the market. Then, one hardly hears a peep from them.

B-15 has never been found to cause toxicity or other harm, and it has been widely used for years, mostly in Russia and other European countries, in much the way the Sabin polio vaccine was used for years outside the United States while Americans were forced to get another polio vaccine that never measured up to the Sabin product.

B-15, a water-soluble nutrient derived from ground apricot pits and in crystalline form in rice bran, rice polish, whole-grain cereals, brewer's yeast, steer blood, and horse liver, has been found to be clinically helpful in stimulating the glandular system and in treating impaired circulation and premature aging. It promotes oxidation and cell respiration, and Russian medical researchers say it eliminates hypoxia—the insufficient supply of oxygen in living skin tissue. It relieves symptoms of cyanosis, the discoloration of skin due to poor oxidation, and it flushes the skin.

B-15 is probably the most discussed "vitamin" in the world. It was introduced in 1951 in the Ernst Krebs' pharmaceutical laboratory, which also isolated "B-17," amygdalin-laetrile. Krebs called its product, which was derived from apricot pits, pangamic acid, from the Greek *pan*, "all" and *gamate*, "seed." It also came to be called B-15. But B-15 as a vitaminic name had been used earlier by Japanese research scientists who had isolated a biologically active fraction from the liver and found it had "growth promoting qualities." The Japanese associated their discovery with the vitamin B-complex, and gave it the fifteenth position. In the 1960s, Russian scientists took the Krebs pangamic acid, mixed with calcium gluconate, then added N, N-Dimethylglycine (DMG) as a free radical but active ingredient, and called it calcium pangamate. They reported that it worked wonders as a metabolism stablizer and enhancer. It lowered cholesterol, normalized blood sugar, kept fat from the liver, improved cellular use of oxygen, and detoxified the body from excessive alcohol and drugs. Since it had pangamic acid in it, the Russians thought their discovery was B-15. But the active ingredient was DMG, known to aid the metabolic cycle of fats, vitamins, hormones, and proteins in the body. Maybe it should have been called DMG-15, which is what FoodScience Laboratories says is the active ingredient of their Aangamik-15 nutrient supplement.

The Food and Drug Administration says B-15 is not a vitamin, since it is pangamic acid, a drug, and not a food substance. A vitamin, on the other hand, is a natural, essential substance in the body. DMG, on the other hand, is a nutrient found in food and in the body. It is said to increase cellular functions and to act as a "metabolism enhancer," thereby creating a state of wellbeing in the body, the way choline, PABA, and the essential fatty acids (EFA) do.

VITAMIN C (Ascorbic Acid)

RDA 45 mg. Water-soluble. Anything over 10,000 IUs daily may produce side effects. Vitamin C maintains collagen in the skin, helps wounds and scar tissue to heal, and helps the body resist infections. Vitamin C primarily builds and maintains collagen, the protein necessary for the formation of connective skin tissue. Thanks to its wide promotion by scientist Linus Pauling, it is now well-known that vitamin C fights allergy-causing agents and viruses, including colds. Vitamin C helps metabolize amino acids, activates folic acid, and prevents the oxidation of other vitamins that are helpful to the skin. It is also a "stress" vitamin. The need for C increases with age because of its ability to regenerate collagen, to aid in pigment formation, and to rejuvenate skin in general. Vitamin C is also said to prevent "bags" under the eyes Cigarette smokers attest to having strengthened lung tissue when they are taking from 3,000 to 5,000 IUs daily. Fresh fruits, and especially

173

citrus fruits, and vegetables are rich in C. Natural C is also found in rose hips, green peppers, and cherries.

VITAMIN D (Calciferol)

RDA 400 IU. Fat-soluble. The "sunshine" vitamin. The sun's rays activate a form of cholesterol in the skin, which is then converted to vitamin D. Thyroid glands need it to make hormones. We get enough from the sun, unless we are sick or pregnant, when we need more D. It is found in fish, milk, and liver oils, and most effective when it's taken with vitamin A.

VITAMIN E (Alpha Tocopherol)

It is considered best to start off with about 100 IUs of E and gradually move up to 400 IUs daily, but do not go over 400, although many lovers of E take 1,000-unit capsules two or three times daily. Our new animal-vigor generation needs vitamin E because consumption of unsaturated fats has increased so. E is an antioxidant, and it can prevent cell breakdown. Applied directly on a wound, it can promote rapid healing. It fights the effects of air pollution on our skin, and retards the aging process by preventing oxidation of cells. E prevents molecular destruction that affects skin pigmentation and elasticity. Megadoses are not necessary if the dict includes daily servings of vegetables. E also protects body tissues from oxygen breakdown. It is best taken before meals and at bedtime. The more polyunsaturates in your system, the more E you probably need. Vitamin E is an ingredient in many skin-care cosmetics, and rightly so, since it can replenish skin cells.

About Vitamin E, the *Nutrition Almanac* (McGraw-Hill) reports:

"Vitamin E is helpful in counteracting premature aging of the skin. It is useful to apply vitamin E to the skin in ointment form while taking it orally, because it affects the cell formation by replacing the cells on the outer layer of the skin. Vitamin E also helps counter the gradual decline in metabolic processes during aging. Dry, itchy skin is often part of the aging process; vitamin E ointment is able to relieve the itching."

SELENIUM

This is a mineral that works closely with vitamin E to promote normal body growth and to preserve the elasticity of the skin by delaying the oxidation of vitamin F. It is found in bran, cereals, broccoli, tuna, tomatoes, and onions. Selenium deficiency can cause premature aging.

RNA/DNA

Most people who take daily tablets of 100 milligrams of RNA/DNA claim they feel more energetic, and above all, their facial skin is significantly smoother. Some report that they have fewer lines and wrinkles. With renewed energy, many RNA/DNA users want to exercise more and eat less. It's great that a vitamin can make one not only feel younger but look younger as well. Nutritionists say the secret is in the activation of the enzymes brought on by the nucleic acids of RNA/DNA—the kinds of enzymes you get from raw vegetables, papayas and mangoes.

The body cells of people who are older than forty have less nucleic acid. Dr. Benjamin S. Frank has shown millions how a renewed intake of nucleic acids can shatter signs of aging, can smooth out forehead wrinkles, lighten crow's feet at the corners of the eyes, make facial lines more shallow, and tighten the skin on the backs of hands and elbow while making the skin plump with renewed moisture. Fish, eggplant, spinach, beets, carrots, mushrooms, asparagus, onions, tomatoes, peppers all provide nucleic acids. RNA/DNA is said to dry out the skin of young people who have oily skin. Marijuana also has been found to lower the rate of cell division by diminishing the cell's ability to make its own RNA/DNA.

VITAMIN P (Bioflavonoids)

This water-soluble vitamin is a companion to vitamin C, and is found in the white segments (not the juices) of fruits such as lemons, grapes, grapefruit, plums, apricots, cherries, blackberries, and rose hips. It is essential in the body's use of vitamin C and in keeping our cell cement—collagen—healthy and working. It strengthens capillaries and prevents them from rupturing from the absorption of the sun's rays. We can get vitamin P from rutin and fruits. Vitamin P combined with C works beautifully to stimulate healthful skin.

VITAMIN F (Unsaturated Fatty Acids)

You can supply your body with fat-soluble vitamin F by mixing four or five tablespoons of unsaturated vegetable oils or margarine into your foods daily. Unsaturated oil is more easily assimilated by the body than saturated oil found in solid animal fat. Safflower, soy, corn, and other natural golden vegetable oils provide vitamin F. Avoid cottonseed and linseed oils.

Vitamin F provides oxygen for our skin cells and gives the cells resilience and "hold-together" strength, and it knocks out unneeded cholesterol in our arteries. Vitamin F is one of the best sources of nourishment for our skin cells. Combined with vitamin D, it can supply calcium to the tissues and help convert carotene into vitamin A. Twice as many unsaturated fats would be needed to balance the saturated fats. If F is taken in capsule form, it should be taken with E at mealtimes. Many persons with dry skin suffer from a deficiency in vitamin F. Such a deficiency can lead to acne, eczema, and a slackening of cell-made menstrual and seminal fluids.

VITAMIN K

If you get adequate amounts of yogurt and acidophilus milk (fermented milk) in your daily diet, your body may be able to manufacture a sufficient amount of vitamin K. And if your daily intake of unsaturated fatty acids and low carbohydrate foods is adequate, your intestinal flora will produce vitamin K.

Vitamin K is naturally found in kelp, green leafy vegetables, alfalfa, safflower oil, egg yolks, and cow's milk. Vitamin K from the body's intestinal bacteria is impaired only when one has gall bladder problems—the failure of the liver to secrete bile—high amounts of antibiotics in the body, or an obstruction of the bile ducts. Frozen foods, air pollution, X rays, and aspirin all destroy intestinal flora and vitamin K.

Vitamin K is essential in blood-clotting, and is often given before and after surgery. It also helps maintain normal menstruation and prevent associated cramps.

Vitamin K can also postpone body and skin aging. It is sometimes called the "longevity vitamin." It is essential for a healthy body and healthy skin. It prevents discolorations of the skin, caused by minor bruises.

ZINC

Zinc is an essential trace mineral with a variety of functions, among which is the absorption and action of vitamins, especially the B-complex vitamins, in and by the body. It is necessary for tissue respiration and for synthesizing nucleic acids, which control the formation of different proteins in the cell. It also synthesizes DNA, the director of every cell's activity. It works best with vitamin A. In recent years, medical science has learned that zinc is a quick aid in the healing of cuts and bruises, helps get rid of pimples, and above all, produces and grows new cells. It can prevent stretch marks in the skin, abate prostate troubles in men over fifty, and prevent liver damage in heavy drinkers. Only fifteen milligrams daily are required by adults. Zinc-oxide ointment has long been used to clear up skin rashes, pimples, open sores, and hickies.

Always keep in mind that drugs can have a damaging effect on the vitamins we consume. Medical science found this out back in the thirties, although the warning is not as common today. Some drugs, such as diet pills, reduce one's appetite and cause deficiencies through reduced nutrient intakes. Drugs can interfere with vitamin metabolism and synthesis. And in some cases, certain drugs will cause the immediate excretion of certain vitamins from the body. Most drugs are not nutritional, except for those used against tuberculosis, which generally improve nutritional status.

Alcohol consumption certainly lays waste any benefits the body can derive from supplemental intake of thiamine or folacin. Any benefits from vitamin B-12 are nullified if you are taking potassium chloride, phenformin, or para-aminosalicylic acid. Any meeting in the body that the drugs Isoniazid, INH, L-dopa or Penicillamine make with vitamin B-6 will cause B-6 to be the loser, as they are natural antagonists. Niacin's effectiveness will also be impaired if it encounters these drugs. Riboflavin is a definite enemy of boric acid, and aspirin is one of the worst enemies of ascorbic acid, vitamin C, among the water-soluble vitamins. Of the fat-soluble vitamins, vitamin A suffers when it is mixed with mineral oil, Neomycin, Cholestyramine, or alcohol. Mineral oil is also detrimental to vitamin D, as is magnesium, found in most antacids. Vitamin K does not function properly in your body if you are taking virtually any kind of antibiotic or drug such as Phenobarbital. Not only do these drugs reduce efficacy of certain vitamins, their presence together in the body can cause sickness, skin outbreaks, and depression.

ABOUT FOODS AND SKIN-CARE

To quote from Clinique: "No skin is at its best without normal nutrition. But no one food will improve the skin. And no one food is a prime skin offender."

How true!

Many years ago, when Americans lived closer to the earth than to television and supermarkets, the American diet was more nutritious. People took in more vitamins and less calories. It was lower in carbohydrates and higher in proteins. The foods were fresher and had fewer preservatives, additives, dyes, and other chemicals that are staples of foods found in stores today.

There are nourishing vegetables and fruits today, but many were raised in chemically treated soil and sprayed with insecticides; meats are treated with chemicals during processing, too. If a consumer does manage to secure foodstuffs that do not have these additives the consumer may still not know what to eat, when to eat it, how much to eat, and what for. Over twelve billion dollars were spent in 1979 promoting food products to the American consumer. Many people who want healthy skin do not know what foods to eat for what vitamins.

It could be we eat too much, and the wrong things. Maybe any skin condition could be helped if we'd just halve our daily food intake and depend on vitamin supplements, exercise, and the right cosmetics. It would surely make us feel better. And wouldn't it also make us look better? Sometimes I think it would be better for all of us if we would avoid the steaks and chops and monotonous peas and whipped potatoes, soups, and inane lettuce and tomato salads, and resort to eating Chinese food. Most of it is a mixture of everything we need chopped into tidbits. We could always order fruits we want, and take our vitamins and brewer's yeast at home. It's no joke when somebody says, after eating Chinese food, that one burp and they're hungry again. No bloat, and none of that overfilled feeling that makes you rush for Alka-Seltzer. A little bran each morn and everything would be in order.

Diets can often be too confusing and imprisoning for some people—even for those who initially lap up every diet theory that hits the market. Why does healthful eating have to be so complicated? Diets have become status symbols. It has become "in" to be on any one of an assortment of doctors' "miracle" diets. You can break out in hives just trying to follow the diet track. Such miracle diets have changed, and even wrecked, many lives.

A simple dicta like "Stop eating so much" brings the reply, "But how can I get my required nutrients?" Some people do stop eating regularly, and instead gulp down

180

huge quantities of mega-vitamins daily. Then, to upset the reliance on vitamin supplements, comes Dr. Art Ulene with the pronouncement: "I have not taken a vitamin pill in years." The popularity of doctors' diets may have resulted from worries over body weight, ailments, loss of pep, and fear of aging and aging signs. No diet anywhere fits everybody. A woman with prematurely aging skin does not know which diet will surely abate her skin condition. A diet low in carbohydrates is of no particular help to a woman with oily skin if she does not get the right vitamins and minerals for oxidating, activating, and regulating the fatty acids in her body.

I believe that a woman who needs skin treatment would do best to take only sensible amounts of those foods having to do with her skin condition and the health of her skin in general. Chicken livers supply a lot more nucleic acid for skin-cell regeneration than chicken soup does. Fruits supply more vitamin C than a big slice of icing-laden cakes does. Fresh, slightly cooked vegetables supply far more vitamin nutrients than pre-soaked, over-cooked vegetables do. Fresh food is always better for body-cell health than processed foods. Canned vegetables lose more than 80 percent of their vitamin C in processing that includes blanching, sterilizing, and soaking. Frozen vegetables lose 60 percent of their vitamin C in processing, and slow cooking takes away half of a vegetable's vitamin C.

What about people on medication? The fad diets do not always tell them what to do. But persons taking Tetracycline risk losing the effect of the drug if they eat dairy products while taking it. Persons taking anticoagulants must shun eating leafy green vegetables and livers, which have large amounts of vitamin K. Vitamin K is a known blood clotter, or thickener. Patients taking drugs for thyroid hormone stimulation should avoid brussel sprouts, turnips, soybeans, cabbage, kale, and cauliflower—foods that ordinarily contain substances known as goitrogens, which impair production of the thyroid hormone.

Some foods—pickled herring, sausages such as salami and pepperoni, and sharp cheddar cheeses, yogurt and sour cream, chicken livers, and bananas—can force the blood pressure up. Beware of wines like sherry and Chianti, also beer. If you are taking a drug to keep your blood pressure down, these items should be avoided, no matter how good they are for the health of your skin.

Drugs not only interact with food, they also have a lot to do with the way a body utilizes food. Often, drugs actually interfere with the body's ability to convert nutrients into body-usable forms. According to the Federal Drug Administration, "Nutrient depletion of the body occurs gradually. But for those taking drugs over long periods of time, these interactions can lead to deficiencies of certain vitamins and minerals."

We would probably be better off if we would avoid processed foods, selecting fresh foods carefully and cooking them quickly to avoid loss of valuable nutrients, and since we now know the value of proteins in building soft, smooth skin, we should concentrate on those foods that provide protein. Proteins do moisturize the skin by helping to provide a strong, uniform film on its surface, which then holds in moisture and makes the skin feel velvety. Cosmetics containing proteins go far to provide this same result.

Any good petroleum jelly, or any cold cream for that matter, that is allowed to stay on the skin for a while will moisturize, but it's a messy task to not only put it on but to take it off. The cosmetics people blend oils with various natural products that provide proteins, package them in a base or foundation that goes on easily, smoothly, and neatly, and that provide the needed moisture.

The body's cells need constant lubrication in the form of vitamin F, now known as EFA (Essential Fatty Acid), and which can be obtained from cod-liver oil. Estée Lauder's vice president of research and development, Joseph Gubernick, says many of the unsaturated natural oils are beneficial to one's skin. These oils—in corn, avocados, peach kernels, and sunflower and sesame seeds—contain a lot of linoleic acid, a fatty acid the body cannot produce, although it is an important skin moisturizer.

"Recent studies," said Gubernick, "show that laboratory animals deprived of linoleic acid in their diet lose an abnormal amount of water. That's one reason we use a lot of these unsaturated oils in our products."

In a 1979 copyrighted Washington *Post* story, Dr. Arthur Upton, director of the National Cancer Institute, had this to say about the proper diet for the skin: "The exact role that diet plays remains unclear." Dr. Upton added that the most prudent diet is a low-fat one, which most authorities advise helps prevent heart disease, but with extra fiber, found in fruits, vegetables, bread, and cereals. He warned sternly against drinking too much alcohol, and added that "too much is more than two drinks a day."

CHAPTER IX

YOUR REGIMEN FOR A
WRINKLE-FREE SKIN

Looking younger than I am is the living end.
Alberta Hunter, Singer

REGIMEN FOR DRY SKIN

MORNING

Step 1. To remove every trace of dirt, cleanse with a rich, concentrated cleanser. Remove the cleanser with a wet, clean washcloth.

Step 2. Moisten a cottonball with a non-alcoholic freshener and smooth over the face and around the eyes to remove any trace of the cleanser. Check your cotton ball to make sure there is no residue. Your skin is now ready for a moisturizer.

Step 3. Moisturize with a creamy emulsion. Dot it on the skin and spread it over the face, using smooth strokes with the fingertips until the cream disappears. The moisturizer will hydrate and protect your skin under makeup.

NIGHT

Repeat Step 1, but then wash with a non-alkali emollient soap. Rinse well by splashing your face twenty times with lukewarm water. Repeat Step 2.

Step 3. Apply a rich emollient cream to balance out the skin. This should be greaseless and yet penetrate deeply to relieve dryness. Dry skin needs plenty of lubrication. Once a week, use a gel or moisture mask. You will marvel at how fantastic your skin will look and feel.

REGIMEN FOR OILY SKIN

This troublesome skin condition is not as bad as it may seem, or as bad as some might have you believe. But to make it less troublesome, you might try these suggestions.

MORNING

Step 1. Wash your face with an oil-free, non-detergent soap. Using a complexion brush, work the lather upwards with circular motions. Rinse by splashing twenty times with very warm water, leaving your skin flushed clean.

Step 2. Using a cottonball wet with a skin conditioner, astringent, or oil-control toner, apply on the skin with upward, sweeping motions, concentrating heavily on oilier areas, being sure not to overlook the areas around the nostrils.

Step 3. There are numerous moisturizers on the market for normal to oily skin, but they should be used selectively. An oily skin can still lack moisture. These moisturizers are usually oil-free. If your skin is extremely oily, use an oil-blotting formula gel.

NIGHT

Repeat Steps 1 and 2 from the morning program, but use a deep-cleansing wash with friction granules three or four times a week and a clay or mud mask once a week to remove excess oils and refine pores. The mask removes dead skin cells and impurities. Rinse off the mask. Now moisturize with a light, balanced emulsion cream.

REGIMEN FOR NORMAL SKIN

You are quite fortunate that you do not have a specific problem. But don't forget you do have a job keeping your skin problem-free. Regular skin care is essential. As you grow older, you will tend to develop dry facial skin and lines. So, to keep your skin as lovely as it is now, try these tips.

DAILY

Cleanse the face and neck carefully with a light, penetrating cleanser.

Tone with a freshener.

Keep your skin moisturized with an emulsion. If you keep up the moisturizing day and night, you will keep that smooth look. Remember to massage, exercise, and stimulate the facial and under-chin muscles to assure your contours a strong resistance to aging and dehydration.

REGIMEN FOR AGING SKIN

MORNING

Step 1. Soak a bit of cotton wool in cool water, squeeze, then pour a light cleansing milk on the ball. Next, stroke upwards from the base of the neck, up over the cheeks to the temples, and then around the nose area and over the forehead.

Step 2. To tone and soothe skin, finish the cleansing process by applying a non-alcoholic toner.

Step 3. Use a moisturizing, hydrating cream to lock in moisture. Make sure it is a light cream, as a heavy

186

one will clog. Select a product that contains plant extracts or one rich in collagen.

NIGHT

Repeat Steps 1 and 2 from the morning.

Step 3. Twice a week, use a deep, firming moisturizing mask, rich in vitamins A, D, and E, and collagen. Do not use peel-offs, as they may pull the skin too much. A gel mask is fine. It can be used anytime to refresh your skin. Leave it on for ten to fifteen minutes, then tissue or wash it off. Apply light toner.

Step 4. Use a carefully selected wrinkle cream lightly on areas where it is needed, and finish by applying your night cream, which should be balanced in rich emollients and collagen, to the rest of your face and neck. This will help firm and smooth out lines and wrinkles. It would also be good to try the live-cell cosmetics now on the market, especially those that contain collagen.

REGIMEN FOR COMBINATION SKIN

Skin that is a combination of oily and dry is not uncommon. The chin, nose, and forehead tend to be more oily while skin on the cheeks is dry.

MORNING

Step 1. Use a milky cleanser to rid the skin of impurities.

Step 2. Using a cottonball, apply a refining toner on the T-zone (forehead, nose, and chin). Use a non-alcoholic freshener on the cheeks.

Step 3. Moisturize dry areas with a good emulsion that will hold your own moisture in all day. Makeup will stay on longer and look fresher.

NIGHT

Step 1. Repeat the morning cleansing routine.

Step 2. On alternate nights, use cleansing grains on the T-zone, then apply toner.

Step 3. Use an emollient moisturizer and smooth it on dry areas.

Method of Applying Cleansers: My preference is for liquid cleansers and those that are not "runny." When applying these liquid cleansers on the skin, rotate with the fingertips until the cleanser liquefies. Remove with a clean, wet washcloth and warm water.

Method of Applying Astringents and Freshners: Saturate a cottonball with liquid and firmly stroke upwards, under the chin, up to the ears and temples, across the entire throat area, then around the nose and up between the eyes and across the forehead. During the upward motion, press lightly on the face while puffing out the cheeks. Lift the lower eyelids tightly, using muscle control, and gently trace under the eyes.

METHOD OF APPLYING CREAMS

Face Cream: Purse lips, and using both hands, smoothly stroke with upward motions. Start from the chin, and work your way over nose, between the eyes, and over the forehead. A small amount goes a long way. If you apply too much, you may clog the pores. Your skin will only absorb as much as it can and needs. If, after a few minutes, there is any cream remaining on top of the skin, blot it off with a tissue. Remember to remove makeup and creams using the same strokes and motions.

Throat Cream: Place the tips of the fingers of your left hand firmly on left collarbone. Use your right hand to apply the cream, stroking upward ten to fifteen times on the left side of the neck. Then reverse the action on the opposite side until the cream disappears.

Eye Cream: Fingerpat lightly, using your ring and index fingers alternately on the area around the eyes. Then, very lightly stroke under the eyes from the outer to the inner corner toward the bridge of the nose. Smooth over the brow bone only. In a few minutes, your body heat will liquefy the cream. Use a very small amount of eye cream and never apply closer than a quarter of an inch under the lower lid.

Applying Soap or Water-Activated Cleanser: Wet your face and hands, work into lather in the palms of your hands, and work with circular, upward motions into the skin. A complexion brush may be used in the same way. This also helps remove dead skin cells.

EVERYTHING YOU WANTED TO KNOW
ABOUT SKINCARE
(BUT WERE AFRAID TO ASK)

Are Gel Suntanners Bad for the Skin?

Certainly not. They are great for people who want a makeup tan without lying or sitting in the sun. Some of the products, such as Clinique's Bronze Gel Makeup, preserve the skin well. Clinique's product is unscented and contains no alcohol.

Is There a Difference Between Sensitive and Delicate Skin?

Quite a difference. Some people think they have sensitive skin when actually they have "delicate" skin. And an " allergy-sensitive" skin is something different altogether. Very thin skin is delicate, often so much so that you can almost see through it. Sensitive skin is sensitive to the touch and to almost anything you put on it. Of course, allergic skin reacts only to certain substances. Know your skin intimately and select products for it carefully. All products do different things on different skins.

Is Electrolysis The Only Care for Broken Capillaries?

It appears to be the only quick way. It costs from fifty to two hundred dollars. Excessive heat causes broken capillaries as does the sun, in fragile skin. Of course, those blood vessels and capillaries could be strengthened if (1) a safe sunblock were used before exposure to the heat and sun, and (2) the body has been fortified with sufficient amounts of vitamins C, P, pantothenic acid, and choline.

Won't Some Eye Creams Make the Eyes Puffy?

They all will, if you don't use them properly. If the substances are allowed to get into a corner of the eye and impact a tear duct, look out for the reaction— swelling around the eye. Eye creams should be gently patted on, starting at the outside corner under the eyes and moving across with gentle pats toward the bridge of the nose, leaving about a quarter of an inch clearance from the lower eyelashes. In the upper area, apply the cream only to the bony protusion between the eyebrows. Use only a tiny amount, as body heat thins the cream and makes it spread.

At What Age Should I Begin Facial Exercises?

When you stop tussling, grappling, tugging, smooching and doing other "horseplay" things of childhood and youth—things that exercise the skin, muscles, and blood vessels of the neck and face. If you stopped doing those things long ago, take note that facial exercises should be undertaken daily between the ages of thirty-five and forty, about the time the skin begins to "relax" and "settle" into a slight sag. If you do them religiously, you'll notice the difference in about four to six months. Firmness you lost years before will come back, and so will smoothness. Your face won't be perfect, but it definitely will look younger. But don't get so happy that you let up. Keep at it no matter where you are. They can be done any time of the day or night.

Should Baby Oil Be Used on an Adult's Skin?

By all means, yes. It's a fact that more adults than babies use baby oil. It's great for removing mascara, eye makeup, and for those dry spots around the eyes. It relaxes tired facial muscles and moisturizes, restores softness, and is one of the cheapest and best skin-care products available.

Will Sleep Create Wrinkles?

Hardly. It is believed without foundation that people who frown in their sleep create frown wrinkles. About all their frowning does is exercise the forehead. Sleep is not only good for the body but for the complexion and a wrinkle-free, puffless facial skin.

How Is Vitamin E Used on Wrinkles?

Simply break open a 400 IU vitamin E capsule and rub the contents on the wrinkle, night and morning. Or sprinkle a few drops of vitamin E into a quarter of a cup of light sweet dairy cream, and add one egg white, mix well, pat it on the wrinkled area, and let it dry for about half an hour. Then wash it off with lukewarm water. Do this daily, if you can, for a month. You should notice a big difference. Many facial creams, night creams, and night lotions contain vitamin E anyway. You can make your cream with as much vitamin E as you want, if you don't prefer the direct approach.

How Can Brown Spots Be Covered?

There are many flaw concealers on the market, which, if applied before a foundation, can give you a flawless look. Just apply after your moisturizer is set, gently patting the concealing lotion over the brown spots and broken capillaries until a smooth look is obtained. Let set and then apply your foundation.

What's The Best Way to Apply Foundation?

I suggest a cosmetic sponge. Wash out after each use. Make sure your hands are clean. Pat over your face and smooth with sweeping strokes under your chin line to blend with the neck. Remember, makeup is always blended with downward strokes, over pores, directly opposite to the way treatment products are applied; they are applied upward, with the little hairs lifted so it can penetrate through the pores.

What Is Pregnenolone Succinate in Formula 405?

Some moisturizing lotions and creams contain very special ingredients formulated by chemists in the manufacturers' own labs, and purportedly do very special things. Formula 405, from the Doak Pharmaceutical Company, was originally created for dermatologists' patients, and contains Pregnenolone Succinate, a patented moisturizing ingredient formulated by Dr. Frank P.

Panzarella, biochemist-president of the Doak firm. The company claims that the ingredient makes its deep-moisturizing product unique. It does, even if just because of the claim. Some Formula 405 users say, however, that the product does help "plump out those little premature lines and prevent new ones from appearing."

Can a Foundation Correct Sallowness?

Yes, if when you apply it you can remember to act a bit like an artist in mixing the colors. For sallowness, try a moisturizer with a tint already in it. This helps you to build your own skin hue before makeup is applied. For an olive skin, use a mauve tint. For a sallow skin, use a red or apricot tint. For a ruddy or reddish skin, tone down with an aqua tint. These tinted moisturizers come in cream or liquid form.

What's a Good Way to Hide Wrinkles?

In some cases, makeup does not hide wrinkles, but rather accentuates them. But try this. After your moisturizer has set, take an eyeliner brush, dab its tip with a small amount of flaw concealer and apply it into the wrinkled area. Let it set for a few moments and then pat the area lightly with your fingertips until it is even with the rest of the skin. Apply foundation, smooth on blush, then, with a cottonball, pat loose powder all over the face. With the other side of the cottonball, puff downward until the powder is smoothed and the skin looks polished. This procedure takes a little time but is well worth it for a smooth look, however temporary.

What's the Best Way to Apply Temporary Wrinkle Lotions?

Products such as Elizabeth Arden's Bye-Lines, De-Markoff's Lotion for Lines, and Imperial Formula's Wrinkle Concentrée must be applied under makeup. Just spread a drop or two evenly over your face and leave it for about five minutes. Good for a smooth look.

Some of these lotions are more of a treatment than a temporary developer. In any event, they must be applied sparingly to a clean skin, and allowed to set for about ten minutes before a moisturizer is applied. After the lotion has set for about five or ten minutes, makeup can be applied.

Is There a Difference Between Fresheners, Toners, and Astringents

These three names are often used for basically the same product. Actually, only the inner layer of skin can tone, and that kind of toning can be generated merely by facial muscle exercise. A refreshing feeling is often incorrectly called toning. Some fresheners contain a cleansing agent, which is quite often alcohol. With the addition of alcohol, these cleansing fresheners are able to get down into the pores and clean them better, cleanse out grease that plain water skips over. And since alcohol evaporates so quickly, it leaves the face with a smoother feeling, especially if the alcohol has successfully removed flaky surface skin. After the alcohol evaporates you feel cool and refreshed, like a man feels after he uses an after-shave lotion. Fresheners with a high alcoholic content are often called astringents. Some nurses make their own freshener-toner-astringent lotions by mixing one part rubbing alcohol with three or four parts water.

The real difference between the packaged fresheners and astringents is the amount of alcohol each contains. Skin freshener is usually 0.1 percent alcohol, and thus suitable for dry skin. The astringent usually is about 0.4 percent alcohol, and better for oily skin.

A toner is generally another name for a freshener and or an astringent.

Do Moisturizers Really Lubricate?

In a way, yes, but they also soften, smooth, and firm. Some lubricant moisturizers found in fresheners cling firmly to the skin, giving it a smooth, soft feel, and are thus "conditioners." The action is similar to that of fabric softeners.

If My Skin Is Smooth, Why Should I Moisturize?

As a precaution, first, and as a supplement to your natural qualities, second. Your sebaceous glands slow down as you age, so any help you can give them before that time is protection against when they do.

Is It Necessary to Use Moisturizers in Humid Weather?

Not really. The skin itself absorbs the moisture in humid air, but you can use your own moisturizer to play doubly safe.

What Is the Best Base Makeup for Winter?

Unless your skin is oily, try using a creamier makeup. Use an oil-based foundation. Do not use dry powder blushes. Gels, cream rouge, and creamy blushers work best over creamy foundations. To test for oil-base quality, put a drop of the makeup on the back of your hand and hold the hand under water. If the water beads up, the foundation is oil-based.

What Type of Cleanser and Moisturizer Are Best for Winter?

If you live in a colder climate and if you have *dry skin*, use a wash-away cleanser. Rinse it off with cool water with no soap. Use a heavy moisturizer during the day. Use several brands so your skin won't get used to only one brand—unless you want to be "married" to that brand. Use a lighter moisturizer at night. Be careful that you don't get it into your eyes, it can irritate and puff. For *oily skin*, use a cleanser labeled for "normal" skin and a light moisturizer during the day, none at night. If the sun gets hot in your area during the day, even during winter months, use tissues to blot off perspiration and excess oil from your face, and take time out to apply skin cleanser periodically. Don't despair. Take it cool, and don't rub your cleanser in. Pat it on.

Is Petroleum Jelly a Good Moisturizer?

It must be, for women have been using Vaseline and other petroleum jellies for years for that purpose.

Is Collagen Good Alone?

It is, but its use alone does not suffice, generally, for what people normally desire from it. You can buy bulk containers and small purse vials of collagen at health stores. It is a grand facial lubricant. You can dab it on any time of the day wherever you are. You can also get your doctor to give you collagen injections.

Can We Overclean Our Skin?

You can overdo anything. Some women have been frightened so horribly about oily skin that they spend hours each day washing and cleansing their faces. This creates a rather raw, underprotected skin surface, perfect for germs, dirt, and other impurities that can cause all kinds of skin damage. It's far better to dab off excess oil and perspiration several times a day, while keeping as much of our makeup intact as possible. A wash in the morning and one at night should be sufficient.

Must Skin Get Worse Before Getting Better?

Only in rare cases, and usually in those cases it's because of the skin-treatment product the person is using. For some people with oily skin full of blackheads and blemishes, a product can produce good results at once, but then two or three weeks later, a backlash can take place: more blackheads and blemishes. Treatment manufacturers say this shows the treatment is working and that after those deep-set troubles are brought to the surface, permanently clear skin will result if you continue using the product regularly. Basically, your skin is getting used to an alien product. Lancôme's Contrôle for oily and problem skin causes some bad reactions in skin beset with acne or sunburn. The company admits this, and also admits that when a customer begins using Contrôle, "breakout may occur at first, but skin will improve and breakout will stop after continual use."

Are There Non-Alcoholic Fresheners?

Fortunately, yes, since some people with ultra-dry skin complain that alcohol is too strong for their super-sensitive skin. Lancôme's Tonique Douceur freshener is non-alcoholic, contains rose water, glycerine, sodium borate, and sambucus, which cools and freshens while cleansing. Sambucus is an extract from the honey-scented flowers of the Elder tree. It is mildly astringent and makes the skin feel soft and clean. It is often used to scent lotions. The Elder flower, however, causes the skin to perspire, reducing body water.

Do Some Facial Masks Cause Irritation?

They do if they contain too much of the aromatic ingredients. Whether the mask is of the hardening or nonhardening variety, if it is overladen with aromatics, the stuff can penetrate the inner layer of the skin and rupture small blood vessels, making them exude, or leak. Mint is highly aromatic, and I know one cosmetic line that has a lot of mint in its products. I'd stay far away from a masking product with mint and other aromatic spirits, or anything that cools for too long.

Does Excessive Cigarette Smoking Cause Lines?

In time, yes. But it has to be a lot of smoking over many years to cause heavy, permanent lines. Smoking coupled with excessive exposure to the sun, heavy drinking, poor nutrition, and lack of facial exercise can cause lines. Cessation of smoking will help erase lines, if other skin-care treatment is undertaken. Smoking can cause so much damage inside the body that it is reflected on the skin of the face, if plenty of vitamin C is not taken regularly. It takes a combination of things to cause lines and wrinkles, and a combination of things to treat them.

Is Greasy Makeup Dangerous?

Anything as hard to remove from your skin as greasy makeup has got to be dangerous. It makes you abuse your skin as you try to get it off. Rubbing stimulates, for sure, but too much rubbing is harmful. Exercising the muscles of your face is fine, but keeping your head in your hands—or your chin on your palm while your elbow rests on a desk or a table—is bad, as it tightly compresses your cheek and chin muscles, cutting off circulation and mashing skin cells together. Always use only a minimum amount of makeup, and even then use a kind that is easy to remove. The more you care for your skin, the less makeup you'll need anyway.

Every woman has what she feels is a flaw or minor or serious condition she feels should be covered up. That's why makeup is so popular.

The I. Magnin Company sells its own I. Magnin Makeup Remover & Skin Treatment, a very effective water-soluble makeup remover with deep-cleaning properties. It is a unique product that helps clear and tone the skin; it contains panthenol for therapeutic effect and the B-vitamin pantothenic acid to aid in healing.

Which Soaps are Best, Acid or Alkali?

Acid soaps are always better. Most soaps are heavily alkali-based and incompatible with the skin of most people, which is chiefly acid. People who care for their skin, and who find it hard to avoid alkali soaps, should keep a bit of cider vinegar around, so that after each face-washing with their alkali soap they can rinse with a water and cider vinegar solution. Max Factor has long turned out a good line of cosmetics attuned to acid-skin needs.

Is There Any One Thing That Causes Wrinkles?

If there was one thing, there would be a cure for wrinkles. Thousands of skin-care people would go out of business overnight. But just as it takes time and a combination of conditions to produce wrinkles, it takes time and many practices to abate and prevent them. And if a person is genetically prone to facial wrinkles, nothing short of a biochemistry miracle will help.

Are Natural Products Best for the Skin?

This question is asked over and over, probably because proponents of natural cosmetics frown on synthetic and chemical products. Everybody says his or her formula is better than somebody else's, but the "naturalists" and the chemical people want the same thing—money—from you. Anything from the soil or ocean is naturally a part of us, since we are all children of Mother Earth, but not everything from the soil is beneficial or compatible with all of us. Some people respond well to laboratory cosmetics, bought in cosmetics stores. Some people find that salad dressing is as good or better for their skin than Oil of Olay. Again, to each her own.

A Lotion or Surgery for Sagging Jowls?

Exercise, replenishing, and vitamins could help, but not at once or forever. A face lift removes jowls, removes and redistributes sagging skin, and surgically reinforces sagging facial mausculature. While a lotion will do none of this, it can help mask, cover, or temporarily smooth out fine facial lines.

Can an Improper Diet Cause Depression?

Most definitely. But both an improper diet and depression can cause bad skin. Every disorder from within begins to show on our exteriors, in some way, in time.

Is Chewing Gum Exercise for the Face?

Very much so. It also helps mental timing and concentration. Gum-chewing definitely exercises the chin, cheeks, lips, and neck muscles. Prizefighters, musicians, and baseball players can attest to that. It's a pity our current social morés frown on public gum-chewing.

What's a Good Test for Choosing Makeup Color?

Put it on, step back, and fold your hands into an X across your chest. If your face, throat, hands, and arms look about the same color, your choice of color is the right one.

Aren't Clay Masks Too Harsh for Exfoliation?

For people with extra-dry skin, possibly they are, but that only applies to ordinary clay masks. Some firms make specially emulsified clay-in-cream mask ingredients, like Ultima II's C.H.R. Creme Masque Concentrate. There is clay in it, and it is the substance that causes the mask to draw and tighten, to stimulate the skin and to slough off dead skin cells that do not rise uniformly but in spots and patches on dry-skin areas of women after menopause. The cream in C.H.R. acts as a buffer, modifying the action of the clay.

Do All Blue-Eyed People Have Problems with Dry Skin?

No. Most blue-eyed people with fair, fine, fragile skin often have problem with dry skin. But some blue-eyed people have olive or tan complexions, and skin that is slightly oily and moist yet beset with other problems such as allergies. In some such cases, the skin will not tolerate mineral oil or petroleum jelly, but does fine with coconut oil.

Is Cold Cream a Good Cleanser?

Some show people say it is tops, but even they admit that while cold cream is good for removing sticky makeup, cold cream itself is too sticky and more than likely to leave dirt embedded in pores and sediment from the cold cream on the face. Then it defeats its purpose. Cold cream is alright as a cleanser if you use soap and water or chemical cleansers after.

Aren't Abrasives Best for Cleansing?

Yes, if you want your skin to stay raw all the time. And there *are* a lot of people who think abrasives go deep down into their skin and while ridding them of dead skin cells uncover an absolutely new person underneath. Heredity, age, and diet are still there. I really do not like to recommend *any* abrasive skin-care cosmetics, as each product has so many "don'ts" and "be carefuls" that effective use is doubtful if not hazardous. I'd rather leave skin abrasion to the dermatologists.

What Is the Best Water Temperature for Washing?

I know some cosmetics people say to use hot water, as Erno Laszlo does in some cases. Some say cool water is best. Some even say cold water. I believe that water that is the same, or very, very close to the body's temperature—lukewarm—is best.

Can Freckles Be Lightened Temporarily?

Yes, with lemon juice and baby oil.

How Can Makeup Minimize Puffy Eyelids?

To minimize, stroke on brown or charcoal eyeshadow, blending well. Then apply a lighter-colored eyeshadow such as white, soft yellow, or pink directly under the eyebrows, blending smoothly. This draws attention to your eyes and not your eyelids.

What Is the Best Way to Make Up Under-Eye Bags?

Light colors heighten and darker colors diminish. Camouflage under-eye bags by applying a darker shade of foundation or under-eye concealer directly on the pouches. Then apply white makeup directly under the pouch. Blend carefully. Let set. Then apply your regular skin-tone foundation.

Should Pressed Powder Be Applied Over Makeup?

A pressed powder is perfect for touchups, but a loose powder is best for setting makeup. It is light and fine and great to slip over foundations.

Why Does Pressed Powder Change Color?

It happens when you don't clean or change your puff often enough. Every time you use your puff to touch up your face, you increase oil and sediment buildup on the puff. This then gets into the powder and darkens it. Sometimes it's wise to turn the puff upright when replacing it in your powder container or compact.

Which Is the Best Type of Mascara?

It doesn't matter what or which type you use, cake, automatic dispenser (liquid), or cream. They all work fine if applied properly. Lashes should be clean and completely dry. Stroke mascara on lashes and let it dry. Then apply another coat and allow it to dry. Lashes may clog if coats are put on thickly all at once. If using a liquid automatic dispenser, remember never to "pump" the brush. You're only pumping air into the container. It is best to twirl the brush gently, then twirl it back into the dispenser. Never use a mascara for longer than three months. Bacteria builds up.

Is There a Best Way to Remove Eye Makeup?

For me, the best way to take off eye makeup that's water-proof is to use an oil-based eye-makeup remover in liquid or gel form. For other kinds of eye makeup, milky cleansers are good. Use Q-Tips, working down over the lids, lashes, and undereyes. Eye-makeup remover pads are also an excellent and convenient method for removal.

Is Yogurt Good for a Facial?

Ideal, I feel. You can make a mask of your favorite flavored yogurt by mixing the yogurt with milk or dairy cream. Spread it lightly on your face and neck, keeping it out of your eyes. Let it dry and remain on the skin for about half an hour, then rinse it off with lukewarm water. It makes the skin feel toned, and refines the skin pores.

POSTSCRIPT

Toward a New Age in Skincare

Women today are living longer.

The largest age group in the United States is middle-aged.

Women today are moving into middle age not with an attitude of depressed resignation, but with a vigorous youthfulness. They are thinking young and doing their best to act young. They are trying to keep attuned to new revelations in physical fitness and are placing faith in science's universal promise of great and wonderful things to come in our lifetime.

But women still fear aging. Above all, they dread the outward signs of it. And well they should. Why must their faces appear to be road maps of their lives? If medical science can make women live longer, shouldn't it also be able to make them look younger for longer?

In a world where a premium is placed on youth and the fresh, unblemished look of youth, countless women are finding it difficult to get their faces to look as young as they would want them to. The warning is *"Don't look old!"* At no other time in our history has there been evidence of so great a save-your-skin quest as is going on today. The search for remedies is enormously extensive and expensive. Cosmetics counters everywhere have expanded, and all offer innumerable

206

and magical new products for the skin, at prices to fit any pocketbook, problem, or ego.

Cosmetics salespersons and skin-care consultants are meeting people from all areas. The expressed problems are all quite similar. But the astonishing fact is that so many women today are coming right out and saying exactly what they want new products to be able to do for them. If the sight of a new facial line or puffiness under the eyes spurred them out of their homes to seek a remedy, they want a remedy, not a dainty new fad in a jar. If premature signs of aging have sent them to the cosmetics counters in a panic, these women want anything they can find to stop the aging in its tracks. They demand something to reverse the signs of the aging process.

And that is where the fine line is drawn.

Where cosmetics people would at one time sell such women a single item, they now offer them an entire program. They also offer them the regular "props," the "hiding-quality" makeup, tanners, and flaw concealers, even the newest in temporary wrinkle removers—anything that might help those offending lines take a visual holiday and just possibly vanish altogether. They are told that some of the items can, in time, do just that.

All of us grow older. Aging is a necessary part of life's ongoing process. But we all must agree that the side effects, and especially the visible ones, do not have to be an attendant part of aging. We have learned that medical science is fighting aging by looking more closely into our bodies to determine what makes us age. We have learned that poor cell regeneration and losses of protein and collagen can and do cause us to look older, often at the prime of our lives, making some women at thirty-five look more aged than other women at sixty.

Can cosmetics help this?

Help, yes. Cure and prevent, no. There are many physiological and psychological conditions that affect our bodies daily and that are soon reflected in our faces. If somebody could show us one factor that causes facial signs of aging and other skin problems. Life would take on a simpler tone at once. If one vitamin could stop all stress, if one set of facial exercises could prevent and erase sagging cheeks and chins, if one diet could make us look twenty years younger, and if one miracle cosmetic could instantly or in time transform our tired faces permanently into a portrait of youth, we could all proclaim joyfully that we had at last found Heaven on Earth.

Today, good skin-care is a necessary process of physical and mental treatment for the inside and outside of the body. If what goes on inside our bodies can cause unwanted developments in our facial skin, then surely skin treatments alone cannot do all the remedying. Just as good skin must have the right balance of minerals, proteins, vitamins, and moisture, so must the body get the same kind of attention and nutrients. We must start off by learning, if need be from our doctors, just what our bodies lack, and what harmful things we are getting too much of.

Cosmetics chemists are working closely with medical people to come up with new products that can be applied to the skin. Recently, they have found that many skin remedies found to be helpful through the centuries are just what is needed today, in the form of herbal, vegetable, and animal remedies.

There is an increasing need for people to pay attention to nutrition, not only what is advertised as fashionable and slimming, but what leads to satisfactory body and skin health.

Discoveries in this new age of skin-care can do a lot

to help those many persons who are trying to combat visible signs of aging. They can also be of immeasurable benefit to those younger women and men whose skin has yet to exhibit problem conditions.

When one considers the importance of skin-care, the ultimate goal should be a total commitment to a lifelong program of keeping our faces forever young.

Patricia Matthews

...an unmatched sensuality, tenderness and passion.
No wonder there are over 15,000,000 copies in print!